To Muriel Brown, Huw Rees and Betty Tate,
with gratitude

REGULATING RESIDENTIAL CARE

Regulating Residential Care

A Case Study of a Voluntary Home

SALLY SAINSBURY
Department of Social Sciences and Administration
The London School of Economics & Political Science

Published in Association with
The London School of Economics and Political Science

SERIES EDITOR: JANE LEWIS

Avebury
Aldershot · Brookfield USA · Hong Kong · Singapore · Sydney

Published by

Avebury

Gower Publishing Company Limited
Gower House
Croft Road
Aldershot
Hants GU11 3HR
England

Gower Publishing Company
Old Post Road
Brookfield
Vermont 05036
USA

ISBN 0 566 07039 1

Printed and bound in Great Britain by
Kingprint International, Richmond, Surrey

Contents

Editor's foreword

In recent years, within the context of social policy, we have witnessed the growing acceptability of the currency of the term "the mixed economy of welfare". In the rush of social policy analysts and practitioners to adjust to the notion of the desirability of including in the social policy framework the voluntary and private sectors as well as the public sector of provision there has been little empirical study of the implications for client groups or recipients of services, of the decentralisation of provision implied by the greater and, indeed, conscious emphasis being placed increasingly on provision by voluntary organisations and the private market. It is true that there has been some discussion at a theoretical level of the political and administrative implications of the loss of public control and accountability consequent upon such a development. But so far, there has been little concern to document the effect of such changes on those for whom provision is made. Indeed, there is little discussion at all on the question of such control in the social policy literature. It could be argued that recent policy changes may have achieved something if they focus attention on the long neglected subject of control in policy areas where public funds are disbursed to small-scale non-statutory and, therefore, non-accountable bodies. It is the purpose of the present study to begin to address the question of such control, more particularly control in the voluntary sector, and its impact upon care provisions.

The subject matter of the study - the problem of standards and the maintenance of standards in residential care, has attracted widespread interest recently as a result of revelations about the scandalously low standards operating in some private homes for the elderly in Kent, and the disquiet which has arisen with regard to public provision as a result of the documentation of abuse and low standards in some homes provided by the London boroughs of Southwark and Camden. However, it is the contention of the present study that particular difficulties attach to the control of standards in provision made by the voluntary and private sectors - the sectors currently favoured for expansion by the government. Although it is true that abuse and low standards of care and facilities are by no means restricted to these sectors, local authorities are subject to pressures of public opinion through the electoral process, and by the audit and the Social Service Inspectorate. Although it may prove to be difficult sometimes to render such pressure effective, the possibility of controlling standards in private and voluntary establishments remains even more remote, despite the Registered Homes Act 1984, a problem which the Wagner Report on residential homes signally failed to address. [1]

NOTES

[1] National Institute of Social Work, Residential Care, a Positive Choice, London, HMSO, 1988.

1 Introduction

Among social policy commentators and analysts, it has become commonplace within the last decade, but particularly during the 1980s, to focus attention on, and to discuss all aspects of social policy with reference to the 'mixed economy of welfare'. It is an approach which considers the operation of publicly provided services in relation to those of the private and voluntary sectors of provision. Indeed, it is increasingly the case that the private and voluntary sectors are seen as of equal importance with that of the public sector, or even in a position of preeminence, in any discussion of social policy. It is not unusual to find that the touchstone in any consideration of the appropriate location for a particular service is the efficiency of the private market relative to the other sectors, as a provider.

There is nothing new in social policy commentators displaying an interest in services funded from private and voluntary sources as well as those provided directly by central or local government. For example, as long ago as 1959, Richard Titmuss was concerned to reveal the 'hidden' welfare system made available by employers, and to compare their impact on the distribution of income and wealth with the 'overt' publicly provided system. [1] Peter Townsend, in a classic study of residential care for the elderly, compared the standard and types of provision available in private, local authority, and voluntary homes. [2] More recently, Mike Reddin has been concerned to compare private market insurance schemes with state systems. [3] And for some years now, comparative studies of social policy have been undertaken to determine why particular mixes of public, private and voluntary provision are adopted in different countries. [4] What is new is the perspective from which studies in Britain are now being written. In the past, such work often made comparisons to extol the superiority of public provision on grounds of cost, fairness, and efficiency or effectiveness, usually in an attempt to defend 'the welfare state' against those who, even from the outset in the immediate post-war years, never accepted the efficacy of large-scale state incursion into social service provision. An early example was the defence of the National Health Service by Titmuss and Abel-Smith against those who charged the service, even in its earliest years with profligacy, and the encouragement of unnecessary treatment or other provision. [5] Most mainstream academics writing in the social policy field sought not only to defend existing public provision but also to extend it. Championship of the claims of the private market was left largely to those liberal economists who remained outside the post-war orthodoxy of Keynesianism. [6] In recent years, and partly as a result of governmental attachment to the principles of a free market economy, academic social policy analysts have been forced to consider the possibility of public provision as second or even third best in competition with the private and voluntary sectors in a situation in which economic efficiency is the primary consideration, and ideological support for the private market considerable.

Yet, in Britain, the mixed economy of welfare has been in existence for centuries. What is new for the post-Second World War period is the particular political emphasis of government in the 1980s and the scale of the problems created by demographic changes to which social policy has to respond. The changing balance in the age structure of the population has created anxiety about the ability of the public sector to respond adequately, particularly in the fields of national insurance, the National Health Service, and the personal social services.

In the case of the personal social services, it is striking that the <u>growth</u> of the private sector is recent and is largely a response to demand for services by the elderly, and for residential rather than community care. It is a growth stimulated not only by the increasing number of elderly people, but also by the restrictions placed on the local authorities' ability to respond because of the financial controls which have been increasingly imposed on them by central government since 1976. Ironically, a further stimulus to private provision of residential care has been the increasingly strong insistence by government on community rather than residential care since 1962. In origin, the policy was stimulated by anxiety about the cost of the National Health Service, and in particular the problem of maintaining, upgrading, and adequately staffing the large mental hospitals built in the last century, and, by the mid-twentieth century suffering from years of neglect and lack of investment. Rejuvenating the hospitals would have been hugely expensive. And even if it were done, there was the problem of attracting adequate staff to work in remote institutions at a time when labour was at a premium. Initially, therefore, community care simply meant non-hospital care. But confidence in all residential care was being discredited by academic theorists. Bowlby's work undermined the acceptability of residential care for children. [7] The work of others, such as Russel Barton, [8] Goffman [9] and Townsend [10] explored the disastrously negative effects of institutional life on adults. Therefore, it became fashionable for local authorities to give greater emphasis to non-residential care provision than had previously been the case. Although residential care for the elderly continued to be a major factor in local authority personal social services expenditure, the focus of political initiatives had shifted to non-residential solutions to the problems of the elderly. There is evidence to suggest that the increasing emphasis on the non-hospital care of the elderly, as of the young chronic sick [11] is stimulating demand to which the private market is responding in the absence of competition from the financially straightened public sector.

While the growth of the private sector in residential care is new, voluntary bodies have traditionally supplied a substantial proportion of residential care places, particularly for those with physical and sensory handicaps. But voluntary effort within the social policy field has never been seen to be restricted to residential care in quite the way that is true of the private market. For it is curious that although private home help arrangements are alluded to in the literature, they have only recently begun to be incorporated into the planning of social policy in some areas in the manner of residential provisions, though private childminding arrangements are partially incorporated by means of regulation. Despite the long tradition of provision, the voluntary sector has proved to be susceptible to widely changing attitudes among policy makers, analysts and the general public.

In the years following the Second World War the major policy objective for what have since become known as the personal social services, was the death of the Poor Law. That death was proclaimed in statute, particularly in the National Assistance Act 1948, and to a lesser extent in the Children's Act 1948, and explored triumphantly in parliamentary debate. [12] The psychological impact of the death of the Poor Law is difficult to overestimate. Although it is true that it had lost many of its functions, the application of the household means test was a recent memory and the workhouse remained the most usual option for elderly people of the working class who, for whatever reason, could no longer maintain themselves in their own homes. The Poor Law still retained child care responsibilities until these were taken over by the Children's departments of the local authorities in 1948. T.H. Marshall has drawn attention to the crucial difference between Poor Law services which provided a basic minimum for those whose income fell below a certain level, and services available to all, regardless of income, allocated on the basis of need for service. [13] In terms of standards of provision, the commitment of the public sector was now open-ended. Statute enjoined the newly established Welfare or Health and Welfare departments of the local authorities to 'promote the welfare of' the groups for which they were responsible - the blind and partially sighted, the deaf and the hard of hearing, and the 'general classes of the physically handicapped'. The same phraseology appeared in the Children's Act. It is significant that the phrase 'to promote the welfare of' was borrowed from the Blind Persons Act 1920, a piece of legislation which was a selfconsciously anti-Poor Law measure designed to remove services for blind people from the stigma of the Poor Law. [14] Despite the financial problems and shortages of material associated with the years of reconstruction, local authorities embarked upon a programme of 'promotional welfare' albeit with little guidance or idea as to how that might be constituted, other than as the antithesis of the Poor Law. [15]

In the context of publicly provided promotional welfare, charitable effort was in something of a dilemma. Since 1834, many charities had acted as the handmaidens of the Poor Law, sorting out the deserving poor for recompense from their own coffers while consigning the undeserving to the Poor Law and, ideally, the workhouse. Although it is true that many charities, particularly those with evangelical origins did not adopt this role, it was sufficiently pervasive for the term 'cold as charity' to gain currency as a suitable epithet to be applied to the mean and flinty hearted. Indeed, so strong was the attachment between Poor Law and charity in many people's eyes, that some Labour controlled local authorities in the immediate post-war years became ideologically committed to supplanting charitable services with their own provisions.

One of the most extreme cases was that of Coventry which sought the legal right to provide its own meals-on-wheels service directly rather than through a voluntary body on an agency basis. [16] Thus it is important to remember, that although voluntary effort was an acceptable and beneficial enterprise in the eyes of many people, including Beveridge, who stressed the importance not only of the co-existence of public and voluntary services, but also their complementarity (a relationship sometimes insisted upon by law as was the case with meals-on-wheels), for many others, charity had become a term of abuse.

Perhaps it is understandable that in these circumstances the Charity Organisation Society, previously one of the greatest adherants of the 'principles of 1834' should change its name to the Family Welfare Association in 1946. [17] Other charities were wracked with self doubt as their traditional role appeared to be diminished by the establishment of large-scale publicly provided services to which everyone, regardless of income, had access. The university settlements dwindled in interest and initiative; even large well-founded voluntary organisations such as Dr. Barnardo's found their traditional activities no longer in demand, and a crisis of role and identity had to be faced in the mid-1960s.

It was in the mid-1960s that attitudes began to change, and charities became voluntary bodies and, therefore, to be welcomed, rather than objects of abuse. Although at central government level lip service had always been paid to the notion of the importance of the voluntary sector, whatever the party in power, there was no genuine commitment to anything other than public provision, except by default. However, by the mid-1960s confidence in publicly provided welfare was being eroded. In part, this erosion owed much to the work of those academics associated with the Labour Party whose studies, undertaken in part to prove to the political right that egalitarianism had not gone dangerously far as a result of state intervention, seemed to indicate that public provision had done little to redress poverty, inequality, ill-health, illiteracy, poor housing, and so on. Such studies increasingly documented the resistance of the public welfare bureaucracies to pressures to respond to individual needs. Indeed, new charities were set up either by or on behalf of groups who were perceived to have been, or considered themselves to be at a disadvantage to the welfare system. Campaigning charities and pressure groups began to proliferate to change the welfare system in their own interest. [18] In the vogue for participation, old charities such as the university settlements began to revive, as community action became popular as a possible means for achieving radical social change. During the early 1970s, when local authorities became increasingly big spenders in the field of personal social services, pressure from the voluntary sector mounted. A series of reports by Wolfenden, [19] Webb et al, [20] and Hatch [21] sealed the image of charities, despite their recent history, as innovative, participatory and experimental. It became a truism that it was the role of the voluntary sector to innovate, and of the public sector to take over and implement the successful experiments on a broad scale.

This expansionist period in the fortunes of charitable enterprises was reinforced in the early 1970s when the assumed benign relationship between public expenditure and economic growth began to be questioned. At the theoretical level, academic economists of both the political left and the political right began to accuse the 'welfare state' of being the cause of Britain's economic decline. [22] In combination with the financial crisis associated with the rise in oil prices, such analysis discouraged high levels of public expenditure. First, the Labour government in 1976 began to slow the growth in public expenditure, and then, from 1979, the Conservatives began the search for cuts. In doing so, they were said to be aiming at cutting the fat of the welfare bureaucracies, and not services. It was in the interests of maintaining levels of service while reducing levels of expenditure on them that government turned to the voluntary organisations and the private market which, with the absence of large scale administrative organisations to support were held to be economically more efficient than local government.

In its enthusiasm for charity the government had forgotten how dependent upon local authorities the organised voluntary sector had become. Even in the nineteenth century, some charities had achieved financial stability only by becoming agents for the Poor Law - for instance, by providing places for disabled paupers in institutions for the handicapped and receiving payments for this from the Guardians. But by the third quarter of the twentieth century many voluntary organisations, and especially those providing residential care, had become largely dependent upon such fees. Even those engaged in community and less traditional work had become used to receiving subventions from local government, especially through such schemes as urban aid, under which central government support was conditional upon that of local government. As local authorities reduced or withdrew their financial support in order to maintain their own services, central government was forced to devise its own machinery through which funds could be channelled directly to the voluntary bodies of which it approved. However, the schemes it favoured tended to be short term and experimental, undertaken and funded on the assumption that local authorities would step in to take over financial responsibility when government aid ceased.

Despite high government approval, then, funding remains a problem for voluntary bodies. But in the residential care field the situation has been eased of late for both the voluntary and the private sectors, by the willingness of DHSS to fund directly the maintenance fees of residents for whom it accepts responsibility. For a short period, the providers of residential care were able to pitch their fees ever higher, until the DHSS was forced to introduce a ceiling on fees, beyond which it refused to pay for maintenance. [23] Having limited the level of individual maintenance fees, central government has begun to express disquiet about the size of the total bill which social security is now expected to pay for those in residential care and is exploring the possibility of introducing assessments of need for residential care for those entitled to maintenance from DHSS.

Critics of the system have pointed to the failure of government to ensure 'value for money' in terms of standards of care, and the government's response has been the Registered Homes Act 1984. The central problem is the question of control where funding arrangements have produced a startling degree of decentralisation and, as Glennerster has put it, 'plurality of service provision largely beyond the social services departments' control.' [24] Even in the aftermath of the Registered Homes Act 1984, control remains a major problem. Indeed, recent research has suggested that in the case of the National Health Service at least, there is considerable reluctance on the part of the registering authorities to insist on standards, since alternative provisions are likely to be difficult, if not impossible to find. [25]

Control is the central issue with which the present study is concerned. Most of the studies which have addressed the problem of standards and control have considered them separately, indeed almost as unrelated issues. Studies of institutional care have tended to concentrate on description of residential institutions and their care practices. Standards have been the major issue rather than the mechanics of control. If addressed at all, the problem has been considered in passing. An exception, of course, was Peter Townsend's study of homes for the elderly. [26] But even here, although the issue of control was considered and its analysis instructive, the treatment was brief and at a general level, and there was little attempt to relate it directly to questions of standards. Furthermore, it has been customary for such studies to be carried out on a 'snapshot' basis, and even if the intention had been there, it is understandable that the formidable problems which would attach to such a study, would prevent a satisfactory analysis of the relationship between standards of provision and methods of control. It is true that during the 1960s, the problem of control and its relationship with standards of care became an issue with regard to hospitals caring for the mentally disordered and chronic sick. [27] But with the determination to empty the long stay hospitals interest in inspection mechanisms waned, despite a succession of scandalous revelations about treatment in such institutions.

A case study over time, of the type described here, presents fewer of the difficulties associated with the 'snapshot' approach.

It is the purpose of the present study to explore the relationship between a single local authority and one of the voluntary residential homes for which it held responsibility for registration over a period of twenty years. The aim will be to try to determine how and why the nature of the control exerted by the local authority over the home changed during that period, and the impact of these changes on care practices within the home.

NOTES

[1] Titmuss, R.M., Income Distribution and Social Change, Allen and Unwin, 1962.

[2] Townsend, P., The Last Refuge, Routledge and Kegan Paul, 1962.

[3] Reddin, M., 'Occupation Welfare and Social Division' in Jones, C. and Stevenson, J. (eds), Yearbook of Social Policy in Britain, 1980-81, Routledge and Kegan Paul, 1982.

[4] See, for example, Abel-Smith, B., Value for Money in Health Services, Heinemann, 1976.

[5] Abel-Smith, B., and Titmuss, R.M., The Cost of the National Health Service in England and Wales, Cambridge University Press, 1956.

[6] See, for example, the work of members of the Institute of Economic Affairs.

[7] For example, Bowlby, J., Maternal Care and Mental Health, Geneva, World Health Organisation, 1952.

[8] Barton, R., Institutional Neurosis, John Wright, 1959.

[9] Goffman, E., Assylums: essays of the social situations of mental patients and other inmates, New York, Anchor Books, 1961.

[10] Towsend, P., op. cit., also Introduction, in Morris, P., Put Away, Routledge and Kegan Paul, 1969.

[11] For a discussion of the effects of closing wards for the young chronic sick, see Owens, P., Community and Severe Physical Disability, Bedford Square Press, Occasional Papers on Social Administration, 1987.

[12] Introduction and Third Reading of the National Assistance Bill, 24 November 1947 and 5 March 1948 respectively.

[13] Marshall, T.H., Social Policy in the Twentieth Century, Hutchinson, 1975.

[14] Abel, R.A.D., The Identification and Registration of the Blind, 1834 to 1968, forthcoming.

[15] For a discussion of welfare departments, see, Brown, M., 'The development of local authority welfare services 1948 to 1965 under Part Three of the National Assistance Act 1948: a study of the relationship between legislative intention and administrative actuality with regard to the formation of social policy', unpublished PhD thesis, Manchester, 1972.

[16] Brown, M., ibid.

[17] Roof, M., A 100 Years of Family Welfare, Michael Joseph, 1972.

[18] For example, The Disablement Income Group, Mind, Chilid Poverty Action Group.

[19] The Wolfenden Report, The Future of Voluntary Organisation, Croom Helm, 1977.

[20] Webb, A., Day, L. and Weller, D., Voluntary Social Service Manpower Resources, Personal Social Services Council, 1976.

[21] Hatch, S., *Outside the State*, Croom Helm, 1980.

[22] For example, Gough, I., *The Political Economy of the Welfare State*, Macmillan, 1979. And, Bacon, R. and Eltis, W., *Britain's Economic Problems: Too Few Producers*, Macmillan, 1976.

[23] The regulations for those in private nursing and residential homes on Supplementary Benefit changed in 1983. In September 1984, a ceiling was placed on the amount payable to any one resident in such institutions through the Supplementary Benefit scheme.

[24] Glennerster, H., 'The Wilting Flowers of Community Care', *Community Care*, September 12, 1985.

[25] Owens, P., op. cit.

[26] Townsend, P., *The Last Refuge*.

[27] For example, Robb, R., *Sans Everything: A case to answer*, Nelson, 1967. And, *Report of the Committee of Inquiry into Allegations of Ill-treatment of Patients and other Irregularities at the Ely Hospital Cardiff*, National Health Service, Cmnd. 3975, London, HMSO, 1969.

2 Method

The study presented here is an attempt on a small scale to begin to explore the subject of public control over non-statutory bodies in receipt of public funds in terms of the nature of the care bought under those funds. Perhaps the orthodox method of undertaking such a study would be to compare the standards and nature of care of a particular type for a single client group by voluntary bodies according to a variety of different styles of local authority control to determine how far and in what ways different control mechanisms affect the experience and standard of life of those receiving care. Such an undertaking would be not only time consuming and costly, but would also give rise to considerable problems of interpretation: for example, it would be difficult to determine how far control style rather than other factors was responsible for variations in standards of care. Nevertheless, this is the type of study which is required if we are to understand the implications for clients of the moves to decentralise provision which are now in progress.

However, in the absence of the ideal, some progress may be made in understanding the importance for clients of the nature of the relationship between local authorities and voluntary organisations, by means of small scale historical administrative studies such as that reported here. The study arose from the unusual circumstances of access having been given by a local authority to its records of a voluntary association home for which it was the registering authority first under the National Assistance Act 1948, and latterly, under the Registered Homes Act 1984. The records consist primarily of files of correspondence between, on the one hand, the home's personnel, its management committee, and representatives of the Charity Commission, and on the other, the local authority. However, the files also included other important material - details of visits undertaken for the purposes of registration, reports on the residents in the home, correspondence between the registering authority and other local authorities with residents in the home; copies of the charity's annual reports, and correspondence with the Charity Commission; correspondence between the registering authority and other London boroughs concerning the present and future role of the charity; the reports of the registering authority's environmental health officers, and the Greater London Council Architects Department's inspectorate, as well as that of the Fire Brigade; and the financial reports sent to the registering authority by the charity.

What emerges from the records is a picture of the residents and those who cared for them, including information on their occupations and pastimes, their meals, and where they go when they venture beyond the home. The senior care staff - matron and deputy matron - employed by the charity to run the home reveal themselves in their own letters and reports as well as the observations of council staff and the charity's management committee. Residents themselves never make any direct impact on the records. Only in those rare cases when a relative writes on behalf of, or otherwise concerning a resident is there anything like tangible evidence of the existence of those for whom charity and borough worked. And although senior care staff emerge with startling clarity from time to time through these records, other care attendants and domestics who must have had a considerable influence on daily life in the home, remain no more than shadows represented by numbers in reports. Much the same is true of those volunteers who helped in the home on a regular basis, though it is possible to pin roles and names to some of them.

The records in the files cover the years 1969 to 1986. But the earliest reports and letters make reference to events and developments since 1965. Thus altogether, there is retrospective and contemporary evidence covering a period of two decades - a period in which profound changes have taken place in the theory and practice of the personal social services. It may be argued that these changes are likely to have affected the style of control adopted by the registering authority over the charity: it is hoped that where such changes may be detected there will be evidence to determine the consequential implications for care practice.

The registering authority concerned was an inner London borough. It is this factor, together with the period covered by the records, which allows for some confidence in determining the importance of control style to care provision. 1965 was the year of London government reorganisation. For the two decades under consideration here, geographical boundaries were stable. Thus one of the major difficulties of longitudinal studies of health and personal social services since the Second World War is removed.

A similar stability is evident in the charity with which the study is concerned. It was set up as a national charity to provide shelter and training for profoundly prelingually deaf girls and women. From that time until the end of the period under consideration here, its constitution remained unchanged. The charity removed the home to the building in which it was to be housed until 1985, in 1922. Thus there was stability in the location in which deaf residents found themselves, though it was clear that over the period of twenty years, the state of the fabric of the building was subject to change. It was the removal of the home from that location to one beyond the local authority's boundaries which prompted the present study.

Furthermore, there was stability even as to the residents of the home. While deaths were reported over the twenty year period, there were few references to new residents arriving. Indeed, as we shall see, one of the problems faced by the charity was its failure to attract new residents to the home, and therefore, new sources of funding.

In view of such stability, it seems reasonable to suppose that any changes in the relationship between charity and local authority, and in care practice, are likely to arise from changes in the client group, in social policy which helps to determine such relationships and care practices, in the administrative structure of local authority personal social services, and the roles played by those who operate local authority social service provision.

Therefore, exploration of the changes in the relationship between charity and local authority, and in the standard of care provided for residents at the home has to be set within the context of developments and changes taking place elsewhere, and it is this which determines the structure of the rest of the book. First, there is the client group to consider. How did attitudes to the care of profoundly prelingually deaf people change between 1965 and 1986, and how were these changes translated into practice? What were the determinants of policies towards the deaf? Second, there is the question of the type of care under consideration. What was the importance for residential care over these years of the social policy context which sets the climate within which practice takes place, and sometimes the rules according to which practice provision is made? Third, there is the degree to which importance is to be attached to changes in the administrative structure devised to implement policies, in seeking explanations for changes in control style and care practice. And finally, there is the question of how far changes in the roles of those who administer services determine control style and care provision.

3 The client group

In seeking an explanation for the variations in policy response which can be identified in relation to the different client groups of the personal social services, it has become customary to point to differences in their position and status within society. Thus, it is argued, children attract relatively generous responses because unlike other groups, they are not economically marginal to society. Indeed, they are widely perceived as being crucial to the future well-being of society. Therefore, it is not surprising to find that children's services attract widespread communal and political support which finds expression in the higher per capita expenditure made available for children's services than for any other. It is this factor, which, it is claimed, explains the relatively low per capita expenditure by local authorities on services for the elderly, though these services are responsible for the largest proportion of the total expenditure on personal social services because of the large numbers involved. Even though elderly people account for a substantial proportion of the population, services for them have so far acquired nothing like the popular political support associated with children's services, if only because only a tiny minority of the elderly require them at any one time. The point may be illustrated by the far greater anxiety aroused by child abuse and neglect than by the illtreatment of the elderly.

Fear, too, may determine attitudes which in turn may affect resource allocation and type of service provision. For example, fear has often stimulated opposition in local communities to the provision of small group homes in residential areas, for mentally handicapped people. On the other hand, it is often argued that mentally handicapped people are widely regarded as less responsible for their condition and therefore as more deserving of services than the mentally ill. Where groups lack popular support, they depend heavily upon interested professionals to ensure the availability of services.

Yet although the pecking order of client groups undoubtedly exists, its basis remains unclear. The physically handicapped generally appear to be more acceptable to the general public than the mentally disordered. But perhaps this is because in the past, the physically handicapped were less likely than the mentally disordered to be shut away in large, remote institutions. Familiarity may be associated with acceptability. Once all groups enjoy a similar degree of familiarity such generalisations may break down as awareness increases of the variations to be found within the general categories of disabled people. It seems clear that already acceptability is determined, at least to some extent, by behaviour: the more bizarre the behaviour of a person, the less acceptable he or she is likely to be. Those suffering from mild Downes Syndrome and mild epilepsy are likely to meet with a kindly public response. Mild epilepsy will often be hidden from employers with the active connivance of workmates. [1] But what about physical appearance? How will, indeed, how do those whose appearance differs substantially from the norm because of disability, compare with those whose condition leads them to exhibit bizarre behaviour, in terms of public acceptability, and therefore, of public and political support?

But, of course, political support for particular services may have little to do with the acceptability or otherwise of the recipients concerned. For example, many of the beneficiaries of the closure of large scale institutional provision which has been a marked feature of social policy since 1962 have met with little community enthusiasm. Yet governments have not allowed this to deflect them from the policy. The policy of reducing the emphasis on publicly provided institutions and of closing mental hospitals has continued to grind on remorselessly, if more slowly than was originally anticipated, because the motivation to do so was grounded on what appeared to be sound financial reasons - usually a stronger political argument than fragmented popular opposition.

Yet despite the difficulty of determining either the basis or the nature of public perceptions of the acceptability of particular disabilities, and its political importance, there is evidence to suggest that popular acceptability does help to determine types and levels of service support for client groups. Among the disabled, perhaps the most instructive case is that of the blind. When social services were being reconstituted at the end of the Second World War, blind people possessed the best developed and most coherent set of community based services available to any group of disabled people. It is now clear that they achieved this by long-term systematic group pressure, which had the result of improving their popular acceptability. They did this by stressing their employability if aided by training, and thus reducing their marginality. It was for this reason that the Blind Persons Act 1920 not only ensured some meagre financial provision for those who were assumed to be unemployable, but also insisted upon the importance of building up a system of training schemes, workshops and aid for home workers, particularly in the supply of materials and the marketing of the goods produced at home. [2] Yet though a reduction in assumed marginality may have been important in gathering political support for a statutory response to the problems of blind people, it is difficult to believe that it has much responsibility for the relative warmth with which the blind as a group are viewed generally, and the readiness with which help is offered by the general public - however misguided such help may appear to be to individual blind people. The concensus seems to be that the blind are wonderful to manage in the way they do, and compassion, however inappropriate and unacceptable, appears to be evoked generally by the sight of a white stick or a guide dog. Perhaps, at least in part this response is to be attributed to the ease with which we can appreciate the benefit of sight merely by closing our eyes.

The contrast between the blind and the deaf is striking. In terms of visual appearance, the deaf are indistinguishable from the rest of us, and on that score should be highly acceptable. Moreover, as a group, they are among the least marginal of disabled people in economic terms. Although they are largely confined to poorly paid work, they generally both find and keep employment. Moreover, the manner in which they live fails to mark them out from the rest of the community. Generally speaking, deaf adults go to work, marry, raise families, enjoy holidays and leisure pursuits, and retire like any one else. [3] Yet at the end of the Second World War, their services were relatively undeveloped. And since then, local authorities have never been encouraged to provide for the deaf by any groundswell of popular feeling to match the enthusiasm with which services for other groups of disabled people were developed. Such evidence as is available suggests that little is known about the deaf among the general public, and, not surprisingly therefore, that they and their problems are widely misunderstood. [4]

The crucial difference between the blind and the deaf lies in the importance of written and verbal communication in our society. For those who have lost their sight alone, there is very little impediment to the acquisition of speech and spoken language. There is no bar to either receptive or expressive communication. And braille allows the blind to acquire information from the written word and to express themselves in writing. Indeed, modern technology enables the blind person both to write in braille and at the same time to communicate in writing with the sighted non-braille user. For the profoundly prelingually deaf, however, the major difficulty is acquiring, understanding and giving information. Deafness from birth or early childhood delays the recognition of the significance of speech patterns. Indeed, the deaf child is isolated from the comfort and warmth provided to hearing children by customary sound. As a result, the understanding of speech is dramatically delayed in the case of the deaf child. At an age when the average hearing child has a vocabulary of several thousand words, the average deaf child's amounts to only several hundred words. The communication problem slows the acquisition of reading skills, and the problem of a limited vocabulary inevitably compounds the difficulty. It is not surprising, therefore, to find that <u>on average</u>, deaf children leave school with a reading age of between seven and nine years. [5]

Lip-reading, the method of receptive communication on which deaf people depend when they are among the hearing, is a difficult art, and even its most expert practitioners can usually understand only about 80 per cent of what is said to them. Even though the special education of most deaf children in England continues to be based largely on oralism, and therefore, is heavily dependent on lip-reading, in practice, deaf people are generally no better at it than the hearing. A major problem faced by deaf people in exercising their lip-reading skills is their generally limited vocabulary: only known words can be lip-read. Poor receptive communication skills in children often result in the retardation of the acquisition of social skills. Because mental handicap and deafness often share common origins, and because some deaf children are late in developing social skills and therefore, appear to be mentally handicapped, it is still possible, even today, for misdiagnosis to take place, and a deaf child to be mistakenly identified as mentally handicapped. And, of course, in the past, when audiological testing techniques were technologically less sophisicated than they are now, such mistakes were common. The combination of poor reading skills and the considerable difficulties involved in lip-reading result, for the average deaf person, in the acquisition of only the most simplified information. Ours is a society which is heavily dependent upon the spoken and the written word. Even television, which appears to be a visual medium, in pratice is heavily dependent on speech. To understand what is going on on the screen, most deaf people have to invest in such systems as Oracle and Ceefax, but of course, subtitles assume literacy and the additional costs of such systems as Ceefax have to be borne by people for the most part with below average earnings. [6]

However, communication is a two way process: expressive communication is as important as receptive communication. If it is difficult to acquire the vocabulary of spoken language with little or no hearing, the problems of achieving speech which is comprehensible to the ordinary hearing person are almost insurmountable. Indeed, most deaf school-children end a largely oralist education with more or less incomprehensible speech. While it is true that teachers of the deaf, and those who are used to associating with the deaf, for example, because they have deaf relatives or friends, may find it reasonably easy to understand deaf speech, for most hearing people comprehension is difficult, if not impossible. Most deaf people admit that both receptive and expressive communication with hearing people is achieved with reasonable ease only with people whom they know well. For the most part, hearing people have neither the skill nor the inclination to take time to achieve understanding with deaf people. As a result, deaf people limit their discourse with the hearing to areas they know well and in which they are unlikely to make mistakes - polite salutation, brief queries about health, and the weather. More extensive communication is attempted only when it is absolutely necessary and when such an occasion arises, deaf people tend to rely on pen and paper, despite their literacy problems, or on an interpreter. Where a matter is considered to be too personal for an interpreter to be involved - for instance, a visit to a doctor - it is often the case that the deaf person comes away with little or no idea as to what has taken place.

For many deaf people then, the communication problem is limited by restricting interaction with the hearing to the superficial and the safe, or to the absolutely necessary. For real communication and real friendship they turn to the deaf community. It is the communication problem and the way with which this has been dealt, which has determined the pattern of service provision for deaf people. Within the deaf community in Britain, the communication medium is British Sign Language (BSL) which owes its origin largely to attempts to devise a signed system of communication through which the meaning of the scriptures could be conveyed to deaf people. As such, it was developed as a direct translation into sign of grammatical English. Even today, most of those who teach sign, particularly to those who wish to be interpreters to the deaf, are themselves hearing. The signing system adopted by deaf people varies from country to country. In the United States, American Sign Language (ASL) derives from a sign language brought from France by colonists in the eighteenth century. As a consequence, ASL is not nearly so dependent upon grammatical spoken English as is the case with BSL, nor does it depend on finger spelling in the same way. ASL is a fast, fluent, one-handed system of communication, whereas, in comparison, BSL is two-handed and relatively slow and cumbersome. Furthermore, the development of ASL has been aided by its far more systematic use within the education system of the deaf than is true of BSL. In Britain, sign language was the main medium of communication within the special schools for the deaf until the 1930s, when technological developments in audiology and amplification seemed to provide the opportunity for deaf children to participate in society's main medium of communication - speech. Therefore, special schools for the deaf switched from sign language to oralism and thus to lip-reading. Although recent research suggests that oralism was probably never so dominant in schools as has usually been accepted, it is true that in many schools, the use of signs in classroom and playground was regarded as reasonable cause for punishment. As a consequence, sign, so much easier for the deaf child than speech, was used surreptitiously, and 'school signs' developed. Even today, the use of a particular sign may mark a young person out as having been to a particular school. Therefore, many deaf children have left special schools since the 1930s without an efficient medium of communication. On the one hand, few deaf children achieve easily intelligible speech or fluent and accurate lipreading, and anything more than a level of literacy acquired by their nine years old hearing counterparts. On the other hand, most schools have studiously avoided teaching, and indeed, have actively discouraged children from acquiring a systematic method of signed communication. Therefore, on leaving school, many deaf adolescents find themselves unable to communicate with the hearing, and, at the same time, have to abandon their childhood 'school signs' and learn the sign language of the adult deaf community.

In contrast, in the United States, oralism never achieved the dominance within deaf education which occurred in Britain. And specialist provision in higher education has been made, in which ASL is the sole medium of communication. Sign language in the United States, then, has been reinforced in the education system to a much greater extent than has been true of Britain. Perhaps it is not surprising to find, therefore, that it is primarily in the United States that, in the field of linguistics ASL is studied and widely accepted as a language in its own right: it is now increasingly common for language to be differentiated from speech. And among anthropologists and sociologists the deaf community is increasingly regarded as a sub-culture defined by language. [7] It is ironic that the pressure which is currently being exerted on both the British and the American special schools to introduce total communication as the medium of education for deaf children should be regarded with suspicion in the United States by protagonists of ASL, who consider that its widespread adoption will weaken the deaf sub-culture, whereas in Britain it is welcomed by BSL enthusiasts who consider that it represents an opportunity for sign to be widely introduced into the education system for the deaf.

Despite its lack of official encouragement through the education system, BSL has aroused increasing interest during the post-war period, from those working in the fields of linguistics and psychology. Conrad [8] has argued that in its substantial dependence on finger spelling and its close relationship with spoken grammatical English, in its present stage of development BSL may be likened to pidgin-English rather than a language in its own right. Others, however, have drawn attention to the existence of two levels of sign language. First, there is a high diglossic sign, which represents a close translation of spoken grammatical English into sign and is heavily dependent upon finger-spelling. High diglossic sign is used on formal occasions of interaction with the hearing community. However, within the deaf community and relaxing with family and friends, low diglossic sign prevails: finger-spelling receeds, signs become fluent, eliptical, and owe little to the grammatical structures of spoken English. There are those who now argue that low diglossic sign has the structure and grammar of a language in its own right. [9]

The deaf community in Britain is defined largely by the use of BSL, and it is within this community that those who depend upon sign language as their main medium of communication, find friendship and engage in leisure pursuits. Research in the United States suggests that ASL defines a community which, operating on a collectivist basis, socialises its members through all the stages of life, into old age and death, far more effectively than the individualised community of the hearing, to which it stands in stark contrast. [10] In Britain, as in the United States, the focus of the deaf community is the deaf clubs which have been established either with the aid of voluntary societies working for the welfare of the deaf, or independently by deaf people themselves. Understandably, in Britain, the contrast between the deaf and hearing communities in terms of their collective or communal, and individualised approaches to life are not so marked as in the United States. Indeed, this may explain in part why the deaf community has remained largely invisible in Britain. Recent research suggests that generally, deaf people live lives which have all the appearance of normality, but which are, in fact, lived largely within the deaf community.

Thus a number of factors have combined to ensure that profoundly prelingually deaf adults have traditionally impinged little on the consciousness of the hearing community or its policy makers. First, the numbers are small. No survey has been undertaken since 1947, but recent estimates suggest that the profoundly prelingually deaf number anything between 0.8 and 1.5 per thousand live births. Second, the deaf community provides much of the support which its members require. Third, the communication barrier inhibits the degree to which deaf people can effectively press their claims for provision on the hearing. Moreover, difficulties of communication have inhibited the development of any understanding of the deaf community by the hearing and their policy makers. Furthermore, voluntary bodies have developed specialist expertise in dealing with deaf people, based on their involvement in the development of sign language, and their continuing role in interpreting and mediating on the basis of their skill in sign, between the hearing and deaf communities. Therefore, for the most part, it has been considered appropriate to allow the specialist voluntary bodies with their skills in communicating with, and their consequent understanding of deaf people, to continue to provide specialist services for the deaf community, unimpeded by intervention from the statutory bodies.

However, during the post-war years there have been two periods when local authorities have shown some interest in developing specialist services of their own for deaf people. In the 1960s, some Chief Welfare Officers and Medical Officers of Health began to appoint welfare officers with skill in sign language who were intended to develop services appropriate to the promotion of the welfare of the deaf. Such developments were largely obliterated by the administrative and structural changes which followed the passing of the Local Authority Social Services Act 1970. During the 1970s, however, interest in specialist services began to re-emerge and specialist social workers with qualifications in sign language began to be appointed once more in some social services departments.

But for much of Britain, local authorities continue in their traditional reliance upon specialist voluntary organisations to make provision for the deaf. In many areas, the only specialist deaf services are those which are provided on behalf of local authorities on an agency basis by the local associations for the deaf. And throughout the country, almost all specialist residential accommodation for deaf adults is provided by voluntary organisations. Thus, in the field of deaf welfare, voluntary provision continues to predominate. And, on the whole, local authorities which are under pressure from groups able to articulate their needs in speech, have felt little obligation to date to disturb the traditional pattern of provision for the deaf.

NOTES

[1] Sainsbury, S., Registered As Disabled, Occasional Papers on Social Administration, Bell, 1970.

[2] Abel, R.A.D., op. cit.

[3] For a full discussion, see Sainsbury, S., Deaf Worlds, Hutchinson, 1986.

[4] Bunting, C., Public Attitudes to Deafness, OPCS, HMSO, 1981.

[5] Conrad, R., The Deaf School Child, Harper and Row, 1979.

[6] Sainsbury, S., op. cit.

[7] Becker, G., Growing Old in Silence, University of California Press, 1980.

[8] Conrad, R., op. cit.

[9] Deuchar, M., Diglossia in British Sign Language, PhD dissertation, Stanford University, 1978.

[10] Becker, G., op. cit.

4 Policy and structure

While it is true that local authority attitudes towards and policies for the deaf are explicable in large measure in terms of the nature of deafness and the deaf community, these have to be understood within the broad context of social policy in general, and the administrative structure within which that policy is determined and implemented. It is the purpose of this chapter to explore the policy and administrative context within which policies generally for deaf people developed from the immediate post-war years until 1970, and which helped to determine the particular residential provision and the statutory-voluntary relationship which are the main concerns of the present study.

Services for deaf people

Local authority responsibilities for making provision for the adult deaf were determined by the National Assistance Act 1948. Unlike residential care for the elderly unable to live at home, the homeless and services for the blind, services for the deaf, the physically handicapped and the elderly in their own homes were not mandatory until 1962. The privileged position of blind services is to be explained by the fact that the National Assistance Act replaced an existing statute under which mandatory services for the blind had been established, while the requirement to provide shelter for the homeless and the elderly in need of care and protection was likewise a transfer of an existing responsibility - this time from the Poor Law to the counties and county boroughs. The National Assistance Act itself offered little in the way of policy guidelines for the new welfare and health and welfare committees and departments other than to declare the death of the Poor Law and to introduce the idea of promotional welfare as the antithesis of the Poor Law. While it was clear that the new policy involved provision on the basis of need for service, not means, and while it was implied that there was an open ended commitment to level and quality of provision, there was little guidance as to the nature of the services to be provided for each of the categories of disabled people for which the new departments now had responsibility.

At the outset, the existing services for the blind formed the basis for a blue-print. Hence the early insistence on the importance of sheltered workshops, homeworking schemes, and domiciliary visiting. Unlike the services for children, there was no statutory requirement that those for the elderly and disabled should be provided by specially trained workers, still less a specific training associated with the job. Initially many of the welfare officers employed by local authorities were former employees of the Poor Law. While there is evidence that some of them found it hard to shake off the residualist attitudes of the Poor Law, many others used their past experiences creatively to develop the new optimal services. Increasingly, with time, the welfare departments provided employment, often part-time, for the growing number of married women who began to enter the labour market in the 1950s. [1] Skills were developed and expertise was built up through practice rather than training, as welfare officers specialised in dealing with a single category of disabled person. Intense loyalty developed towards the particular set of services within which a welfare officer worked: it became customary for welfare officers to champion the interests of their blind, or their deaf. [2] In the course of the 1960s, specialist workers trained in manual communication - Deaf Blind Manual as well as BSL - began to be appointed specifically to develop services for deaf people. Thus by the end of the 1960s, to occupational specialisation associated with client group, was beginning to be added, in the case of the deaf, a specific communication skill. Such specialists began to provide a local authority based interpretation service, and a source of support and mediation for the deaf community focussed on deaf clubs.

Yet the development of such services remained haphazard and piecemeal. Even after 1962, when schemes for the disabled became mandatory, the level and type of service provision to be made remained at the discretion of local authorities. Even the size of the potential client group in each of the categories identified under the National Assistance Act 1948 remained a mystery. Registration was voluntary, and no definitions were devised by which membership of groups such as the deaf, hard of hearing, and partially sighted, still less of the general classes of the physically handicapped could be determined. The decision as to whether or not it was appropriate for a particular person to be registered was usually left to the discretion of individual welfare officers. Local authorities themselves varied widely in their attitudes towards registration. While most were content to leave registration decisions to welfare officers, by the 1960s there were some which insisted that receipt of service should be conditional upon registration. Still others were content to encourage the collection of names for registers and did little else. The only register which was assumed to be anything like complete was that for the blind: there were agreed national definitions of blindness, ascertained and certificated by approved medical inspection. And although registration of the blind was not compulsory, there were financial inducements for them to register. While it is true that the blind pension for which registration was a requirement, was abolished in 1948, there were other financial concessions to the blind, such as the blind scale rate under the National Assistance (later the Supplementary Benefit) scheme, and the special income tax rate, for which it was essential to register. Moreover, the Blind Register was long established and widely accepted. But studies carried out in the later 1960s by Sorsby and Abel were to show that even in the case of the blind, registration was far from complete. [3]

In the case of other groups, for whom there was no official definition, and, for the most part, little inducement to register, the registers were largely meaningless, either as indicators of the size of a particular population, or of the need for a particular set of specialist services. Indeed there were wild variations between local authorities in the number per thousand population which they registered, differences which could not be explained entirely in terms of variation between areas in the incidence of particular disabilities. Measured in terms of levels of expenditure per annum per person registered, it became clear in the 1960s, that there were substantial differences between local authorities in the level of service they provided for all the categories of disabled people for whom they had responsibility. [4] Even today, local authorities vary in their rates of registration for 'the deaf without speech'. However, in the case of the deaf, both the 1947 national survey and the 1975 estimate [5] suggest that there are considerable regional variations in the incidence of deafness and that to some extent these explain regional variations in registration rates.

The focus of the services being developed for the deaf as for other disabled people, was community and domiciliary based rather than residential. In this respect, local authorities were creating services which, in part, parallelled those of the specialist voluntary bodies. Traditionally, the voluntary organisations for the deaf, had been concerned with helping to ensure the availability of religious services and clubs for the deaf, maintaining an informal interpretation service, and a supply of interpreters, and maintaining contact with deaf people marooned among the hearing, such as those in mental hospitals. Yet much of the effort of specialist voluntary organisations for the deaf as for other groups of disabled people, continued to be directed at the residential care field. Throughout the immediate post-war years, residential care policy for the deaf was largely subsumed within that for the elderly. And it was the residential care of the elderly, which dominated the work of the welfare and the health and welfare departments. Although the proportionate increase of expenditure on domiciliary and other community based services was huge, it took place from a tiny base, and throughout the 1950s and 1960s, the financing of residential care for the elderly accounted for the lion's share of the expenditure of the health and welfare departments.

Residential care

Government policy towards the residential care of the elderly was determined in part, by ideas about what constituted a non-Poor Law approach to such provision, and the prevailing economic climate. Ideally, it was hoped that the large Poor Law institutions would give way to provision which would resemble that bought by the middle classes in their old age in hotels. Hence, initially, great importance was attached to the pension book, which was to enable all elderly people to buy their care and accommodation when the need arose, and the ministeriallly guaranteed allowance which ensured that no one would be rendered destitute in the process. Apart from this, policy preoccupations centred on the size of homes and the desirability of single bedrooms. It was considered that the essence of the Poor Law institution, apart from the insistence on destitution, was regimentation associated with size. Therefore small homes, and the abolition of dormitories were considered to be the hall-marks of a progressive policy.

However, in practice, the rate at which such homes were established, and whether they had single, double, or three bedded rooms, depended upon financial considerations and the availability of raw materials at any one time. In the context of post-war reconstruction and debt repayment, financial stringency was inevitable, while priority for the use of scarce imported raw materials was given to public housing. The decision of the Attlee government to rearm, and Britain's entry into the Korean war exacerbated the difficulty. Even so, new purpose built homes were established, though by the end of the 1950s, as many as 30 per cent of the elderly in residential care were in former Poor Law institutions. [6]

It was this situation which Townsend chose to study at the end of the 1950s. The importance of The Last Refuge [7] lies not only in the fact that it is a superlative piece of analysis and one of the seminal works in the field of social administration, but also that it wrong-footed the government in its view of the nature of community care. Ever since its inception, the cost of the National Health Service had been a matter of political controversy, despite attempts to prove that it was more cost-effective than private medicine. Accusations of the misuse of the service, of patients needlessly wasting doctors' time, and unnecessary claims for spectacles and false teeth persisted throughout the 1950s. And at the end of that decade, the political necessity for financial retrenchment ran up against the problem of the mental hospitals. Most of these institutions were large scale, and had been built in the last century, usually on the colony principle, in remote rural areas, and surrounded by huge grounds, the cultivation of which was intended both to supply the institution with produce and to provide patients with healthy outdoor activity. By the 1950s, it appeared to be anachronistic for patients to acquire agricultural rather than industrial skills, and the farms, in any case, were now sources of financial loss: the Ministry of Health began a policy of land sales. Far more important, however, was the state of the hospital buildings which had suffered from a lack of investment from the outset and which would prove difficult to adapt to take advantage of modern technology and allow savings to be made on financial and human resources. However, their replacement would be prohibitively expensive. Furthermore, their location made it difficult for them to attract staff at a time of labour shortage. Finally the staff of mental hospitals attracted little support from elsewhere in the National Health Service which was dominated by the teaching hospitals, where staff had inherited the ethos of their predecessors, the voluntary hospitals, especially their insistence on the superiority of the cure of acute conditions, and their lack of interest in the care of chronic patients.

The moment was politically opportune for the report of the Royal Commission on mental health, which, resting its case on the desirability of treating mental disorders with drug therapy, urged the establishment of an open door policy which would encourage early treatment and a change in attitudes, so that the treatment of mental disorders could take place on the same basis as that of physical disorders. As a consequence, it urged a move towards outpatient and short term hospital treatment. [8] The Mental Health Act 1959, which gave statutory expression to many of the Report's recommendations, identified as the first priority, the establishment of hostels by local authorities both to delay entry into hospitals, and to provide a half way stage for those returning to the community from hospital.

Such policy changes, which had been promoted largely from political and financial motives, began to be blessed by academic theorists whose analyses of large institutions, such as those for the mentally disordered, questioned for whose benefit they were run, detailed their wholly negative effects on those they were intended to help, and denied the possibility of treatment within them. Therefore, when, in 1962, the government produced its Hospital Plan, [9] and in the following year, the blue book Health and Welfare - the Development of Community Care, [10] it was able to count itself among the good and the progressive. The proposal was to run down the mental hospitals, and increase local authority provision, both domiciliary and residential. It was clear at this stage that, from the government's point of view, community care was any non-hospital care, and therefore, it included local authority residential services. It was this position which Townsend changed.

In fact, Townsend's theoretical framework for his study of residential homes for the elderly, owed relatively little to the influential sociological and psychological studies of large institutions. He relied far more on Bowlby's studies of children both to destroy the viability of institutions as a means of care, and to establish criteria for an acceptable alternative system of care. Townsend argued the applicability to everyone of Bowlby's insistence on the crucial importance for children of love, warm relationships and family. Townsend's own previous work predisposed him to this point of view. [11] His study of the family life of elderly people in East London suggested both an ideal and the possibility of its realisation: everyone had the right to live a normal life which Townsend identified as the giving and receiving of love and services on a reciprocal basis between the generations of a three or four or more, generational family. There was no prospect of an institution which was able to provide 'normality' in this sense. Therefore all institutions should be closed, and replaced by care in the community, meaning care with or near relatives, or, if there was no family, in the midst of substitute families created by domiciliary services and neighbours. [12]

While governments in the 1960s were increasingly persuaded by Townsend's view of community care as non-institutional care, policy makers, in both central and local government tended to see its realisation as a long term ideal. However, for financial reasons there appeared to be a good case for laying greater emphasis on domiciliary as opposed to residential care. But the study was also important at the practical level in creating ambivalence about existing residential care, and in providing criteria according to which homes might be judged as enabling their residents to acquire normality to a greater or lesser extent. Thus the appropriateness of the nursing qualification for those running homes was questioned in view of the evidence that only a minority of residents required substantial help with personal care and other daily tasks. The importance of maintaining links with the family, and encouraging interaction with the neighbourhood, as well as participation in household duties and decision making within the homes began to be stressed. Emphasis was placed on privacy, and the availability of space for personal possessions. Thus changing the regime of homes, delaying entry into residential care became policy preoccupations rather than the removal of residential care as a policy option. It is within this context that the home which is the centre of the present study, has to be understood.

Voluntary homes and local authorities

But how could such policy developments impinge on a voluntary home for deaf women and girls? Townsend's survey of homes for the elderly included homes run by voluntary organisations. Of course, their status as charities was conditional upon their capacity to satisfy the Charity Commission. But the Commission is concerned not with the nature of the care required, or the normality or otherwise of the lives of those in residential accommodation, but with whether or not a voluntary body is fulfilling its charitable obligations. Thus the questions the Commission would ask regarding the home with which we are concerned here are not 'Are the deaf women in the home happy?' and 'Are they encouraged to interact on a social basis with others living in the neighbourhood?' but 'Does the organisation provide accommodation for deaf and dumb women and girls?' and 'Does it do so on a non-profit making basis?'

However, under the National Assistance Act 1948, with some exceptions, those in charge of homes for the aged and handicapped were required to be registered with, and for this purpose to have their premises inspected by the local authority. In practice, however, Townsend [13] discovered enormous variety in the quality and frequency of inspection, and concluded that, in general, the relationship between local authority and voluntary home was often insubstantial. Of the 39 voluntary homes included in his study, two had never been registered, a third had not been inspected within the last twelve months, while six had not been visited for the last five years. Most of the rest (less than half) had been inspected in the last six months. In terms of frequency, a few homes were visited every three months, a few more every six months, while others were visited every twelve months.

The nature of the inspection process also varied substantially from one local authority to another. In a few cases, matrons described a thorough inspection lasting between one and two hours, which involved showing the registration officer around and answering detailed questions about the home. Others, however, described a more perfunctory affair involving no more than a casual conversation over a cup of tea. Whatever the nature of the inspection, matrons resented the interference, and so did the national voluntary organisations 'who suspected the ability and efficiency of the local authorities even when they conceded the principle of public supervision'.

Townsend discovered other methods by which contact was maintained between voluntary homes and local authorities beyond the formalities of the registration process. For example, welfare officers often visited a number of homes when they were arranging to pay the balance of the maintenance fees. Sometimes the Chief Welfare Officer was invited to serve on the committee of the voluntary association responsible for the home. In other cases, relationships established between voluntary homes and local authorities were even more informal. For example, there were cases in which the wives of local councillors were members of the voluntary association's committee; and there were instances in which ex-mayors were committee members. It seems that semi-formal arrangements of this kind were not unusual.

In general, however, matrons and their voluntary association committees were left to face their problems alone, with little external professional advice and support. And the problems which they faced were considerable. Townsend reports that matrons and committee members of the voluntary associations frequently referred to their shortage of money. Indeed, nearly half reported that their homes required either 'material improvements and structural alterations and repairs', such as new heating systems, redecoration, new furnishings and toilet facilities, or extra staff, for which there were insufficient funds.

London government

By the time the file of correspondence on the Home opens, the administrative setting within which the relevant sections of the National Assistance Act were administered had been changed in one important respect. In 1948, counties and county boroughs were required to set up welfare departments under a Chief Welfare Officer, or combined health and welfare departments under the Medical Officer of Health responsible to welfare or health and welfare committees of the local authorities respectively, to administer the Act. The creation of the new departments responsible for promoting the welfare primarily of the physically disabled represents the final phase of the gradual demise of the all-purpose destitution authority and its replacement by specialist services divided according to function in the manner for so long championed by the Webbs. Until 1964, the administrative unit with registration reponsibilities for the Home was the London County Council, which contemporary studies suggest was innovative and expansionist in its attitude to the welfare services. [14] But the considerable unease which had been generated by Britain's historically high but comparatively low growth rate in the 1950s resulted in the conviction that the economic and industrial rejuvenation and modernisation of Britain depended upon more effective planning. The system of counties and county boroughs, established in the last major reorganisation of local government in 1888 and 1892, appeared to be unsuitable for the requirements of modern planning: their areas were too small for the purpose of spatial planning or to take advantage of the economies of scale which would allow for more cost-effective and responsive provision. A difficult tight-rope had to be negotiated to balance the requirements of local democracy and planning. Much was made by the proponents of reform of the low turn-out in local elections, which suggested that existing forms of local government aroused little interest or loyalty: larger areas with greater responsibilities would create greater participation in the democratic processes. [15] The rest of the country had to await the deliberations of its own Royal Commission, as well as considerable political manoeuvring until 1974 for local government reform. But London government was transformed in 1965 by the London Government Act 1963.

The area of London was enlarged to take account of its suburban expansion in the twentieth century and the county councils of London and Middlesex ceased to exist. Their welfare responsibilities were transferred to the welfare departments of enlarged boroughs, which usually comprised the amalgamation of a number of old boroughs, while new outer London boroughs were created out of parts of the counties whose boundaries had been invaded by suburban London. The whole of the new area now designated as Greater London was to have a single strategic planning authority, the Greater London Council, with little concern with direct service provision. Thus the welfare department which had responsibility for the registration of the Home, was a relatively new creation; the borough itself was a recent amalgamation of old London boroughs, and in common with other London boroughs, in administering the National Assistance Act, it was exercising powers which had not belonged to this tier of London government before.

NOTES

[1] Rodgers, B. and Dixon, J., Portrait of Social Work, Oxford University Press, 1960.

[2] Brown, M., op. cit.

[3] Abel, R.A.D., An Invesgitation into Some Aspects of Visual Handicap, Statistical and Research Report, Series No. 14, HMSO, 1976.

[4] Sainsbury, S., Registered as Disabled. See also Sainsbury, S., Measuring Disability, Occasional Papers on Social Administration, Bell, 1973.

[5] Advisory Committee on Services for Hearing Impaired People, Report of a Sub-Committee Appointed to Consider the Role of Social Services in the Case of the Deaf of all Ages, DHSS, June 1977.

[6] For a full discussion, see Townsend, P., op. cit.

[7] Ibid.

[8] Report of the Royal Commission on the Law Relating to Mental Illness and Mental Deficiency, London, HMSO, Cmnd. 169, 1957.

[9] Ministry of Health, A Hospital Plan for England and Wales, HMSO, London, 1962, Cmnd. 1604.

[10] Health and Welfare, the Development of Community Care, HMSO, Cmnd. 1973, 1963.

[11] Townsend, P., The Family Life of Old People, Routledge and Kegan Paul, 1957.

[12] Townsend, P., The Last Refuge.

[13] Ibid.

[14] Sainsbury, S., Registered as Disabled.

[15] Royal Commission on Local Government in Greater London 1957-1960, London, 1960, HMSO, Cmnd. 1164.

5 The Home and the Borough 1965 to 1971

Exploration of the relationship between the Home and the Borough appears to divide naturally into three unequal periods of time. The first begins in 1965, with the setting up of the new London boroughs and the establishment of their welfare departments, and ends in 1971 when the social services departments were established following the passing of the Local Authority Social Services Act 1970. Although the letters and memoranda in the files begin in January 1969, they contain some retrospective evidence for the nature of the relationship between Home and Borough for the preceeding three and a half years.

It is clear merely from the number of items in the records for each of the years 1969, 1970, and 1971 that the borough was by no means adopting the laissez faire approach to voluntary homes which might have been expected from the Townsend survey of homes for the elderly and from what is known of local authority attitudes towards services for the deaf. Indeed, it is clear from the outset that in this Borough, the requirement under the National Assistance Act 1948 'to promote the welfare of the deaf' was taken seriously. In 1969, there were only two months when no item of correspondence was placed in the records. Altogether, there are 25 different items on the file for this year. It is true that such a flurry of activity was not matched in the subsequent two years. But even so, in 1970, there are only six months for which there are no records on the file, and this is true of five months in 1971. For 1970, there are records of eight communications regarding the Home, and for 1971, as many as eighteen.

The number of items involved and their spread throughout the three year period suggest a considerable and sustained interest on the part of the local authority. But even more telling is the evidence given by the correspondence of the range of interest shown by the welfare department. First, there is the question of registration and the reports associated with it. Then there are the reports on individual residents who were the direct responsibility of the borough as well as reports to other local authorities on the residents for whom they were responsible. Other items concern the activities of residents, including their holidays, and their contacts outside the Home. Still others relate to the management and staffing of the Home, its physical structure, and its financial situation.

The registering authority

It is clear from the outset that the promotional attitude adopted by the local authority towards the Home arose from the considerable and direct interest of three people - the Chief Welfare Officer, the Registration Officer, and the specialist Welfare Officer for the deaf. This, then, was one of those welfare departments which was pioneering the development of services for the deaf, beginning with the employment of a welfare officer proficient in manual communication. But it is also clear from the energy with which the Registration Officer pursued her task, that the Department used its position as the registering authority to monitor and attempt to improve the care regime and the lives of residents of at least one of the voluntary homes within its boundaries. The existence of the one or the other alone might have achieved much: an energetic policy of registration combined with frequent and regular visits of inspection could well have influenced for the better care practices in the Home, but without any real understanding of the special requirements of deaf people; a good specialist welfare officer alone could have helped to develop services for the deaf, but it is unlikely that he would have made much impact on the care regime of the Home. The conjunction of the two was of critical importance for the policy which was to be followed over this three year period, and it seems clear that the Chief Welfare Officer was crucial in achieving this.

It seems to be the case that the springboard for the promotional activity of the local authority was the inspection visit for registration purposes, and that this had been taking place, together with the visits of the specialist Welfare Officer since the establishment of the Welfare Department. Early in the records, there is a report by the deaf Welfare Officer in which, describing his own visit to the Home on 9 January 1969, he paid tribute to the effect on the Home of the Registration Officer's visits over the previous three and a half years, to which he attributed the improvements which had taken place there. The registration form itself required answers to a wide range of questions covering many aspects of homes and the lives of their residents. Apart from details of the person or body which required registration, the address, and the type of persons for whom accommodation was provided, the particulars of all staff were required, as well as information regarding the occupancy of bedrooms, the decoration and furnishing of day rooms, and the acceptability of the kitchen offices. Descriptions were also required of bathrooms, washing facilites, and WCs, including how many were set aside exclusively for staff use. Information had to be provided on diet, and the registering officer was asked to check the time of the last meal, whether a late drink was available, and the content of lunch on the day of the visit. Heating and lighting arrangements had to be described, and the officer was required to discover if heating was included in the fees. Recreational facilities for residents were recorded as well as medical arrangements - whether a doctor paid regular visits, whether medicines and drugs were issued by the staff, and whether there was a locked drug cupboard. A description of night supervision arrangements was required, as well as the arrangements for clothing residents. A space was available on the form on which the registering officer was able to record the details of other facilities available at the home. A statement of fees was required, as well as details concerning the exhibition of the Registration Certificate itself, the security of the residence, and the fire precautions in operation. The form concluded with a space set aside for general observations, and another for points 'to be noted at subsequent inspection'. There was also a space in which the date of the next inspection had to be recorded.

To comply with the requirements of the registration form, the visit of the registration officer had to amount to a good deal more than 'a casual chat over a cup of tea'. If the requirements of the form were to be met satisfactorily, a visit of between one and two hours, during which the officer was shown around, and matron was required to submit to searching questions, was necessary. The form itself was printed on two sides of a foolscap sheet of card, and in the case of the Home for the Deaf, the details required were meticulously recorded, closely written by hand.

Although it is clear that registration visits had taken place on a regular basis since 1965, the first for which there are records was that which took place on 9 January 1969. On this occasion, the Registering Officer was accompanied by the specialist Welfare Officer who filed his own independent report of the visit. The first registration report portrayed a medium size Home with the capacity to take 32 residents, though, in fact, only twenty four were given accommodation at the time of the visit. Despite the improvements which were said to have taken place in the previous three and a half years, the picture which emerges is of a rather spartan establishment. It is clear that there was little privacy or room for personal effects in the manner which by then was considered desirable by government to humanise institutional life: beds were divided between three dormitories. The residents had four meals a day, including a cooked breakfast, which were considered to be of a satisfactory standard. The kitchen in which they were prepared and cooked was declared to be clean. There was one bathroom with three baths and 'several basins'. All laundering was undertaken within the Home, and residents were provided with clothing. A doctor called once a month, as did a chriopodist. Cover at night was provided by matron and her assistant.

The staffing and management of the Home

The staffing of the Home was regarded as a problem by both the Registering Officer and the specialist Welfare Officer. Not only were staffing levels considered to be low, Matron herself was seen as a considerable obstacle to change. They both referred to 'matron's restraining influence'. Both comment that on this first visit in 1969, an easier atmosphere prevailed because Matron was sick and had taken to her bed. Despite these difficulties, a determined effort was in progress to use registration visits as an instrument of change. Thus, a visit for re-inspection took place on 15 July 1969, and the occasion was used to check on how far the shortcomings of the Home, noted at the January visit, had been made good. In fact, no action had been taken with regard to the fire notice which had not been properly displayed at that visit, and there were still no curtains at the dining room windows. Matron, who had decided to retire in the following September, was warily described as being 'as resistent to change as ever'. However, some hope was placed in a recently acquired member of staff: 'Perhaps new curtains will be put up now that there is a new gardener/handyman.' The fire notice and the curtains are itemised as points to be noticed at subsequent visits. The information acquired at inspection visits was not merely filed away. After the visit, the Registration Officer wrote a note to the Chief Welfare Officer asserting the need for new wardrobes, stair carpet, floor coverings for the schoolroom and the landing, as well as curtains and lampshades in the day rooms, at the Home. Within two weeks of the registration visit, on 28 July 1969, the Chief Welfare Officer sent a letter to this effect to the Chairman of the Home's Management Committee.

With the possibility of a new matron, the Chief Welfare Officer wrote again to the Chairman of the Management Committee on 6 August 1969, to point out that any such change would require a new registration. The Chairman replied on 4 September that the name to be registered was not yet known, but that the Department would be informed as soon as an appointment was made. Subsequently, on 9 December 1969, the Registration Officer and the specialist Welfare Officer again made a joint visit, to effect a new registration. This time, the decoration and furnishing of the sitting room was regarded as inadequate, and it was noted that the curtains had still not been put up in the dining room. The lack of curtains and the continued failure to display the fire notice properly were again itemised for notice on subsequent visits. The Registration Officer recorded that the assistant matron had expressed surprise at the amount of money available for modernisation, but explained that nothing could be done without the agreement of Matron and the Committee.

It might be thought that the degree of pressure exerted by the Welfare Department through the registration process would be resented by the voluntary association responsible for the Home, and certainly, Townsend's evidence would support such an assumption. But if there was resentment it did not surface in the records. Indeed, there is contrary evidence which suggests that the views of the Department were valued by the Management Committee. This emerges most clearly with regard to the question of staffing. The objection to the existing Matron was not merely that she exerted a restraining influence and resisted change, but more importantly, that she encouraged in staff an inappropriate and undesirable attitude toward the residents. After his visit on 9 January 1969, the specialist Welfare Officer reported of the residents that 'staff see them as backward children'. Therefore, it is not surprising that hopes for change were raised by the prospect of Matron's retirement in September of that year. In the meantime the post of assistant matron became vacant, and the Management Committee sought the advice of the Welfare Department on the matter. On 30 April 1969, the Chief Welfare Officer received a telephone call, asking for advice regarding the type of person for whom they should look when advertising for a replacement. A draft copy of the advert was sent for comment. It was decided to ask for someone with a nursing background and skills in manual communication. Further requirements were progressive thinking and a flexible approach to care. The advertisement was to be placed in a selection of daily, local and specialist papers. It appears that the discussion about staffing requirements took place within the context of a more general consideration of the role of the Home. When, on 11 June 1969, the Chief Welfare Officer sent the final agreed version of the advertisement to the Chairman of the Management Committee, he referred in passing, in his covering letter, to their discussion regarding the future of the Home. Obtaining a new matron proved to be more difficult, but in this case, too, it is clear that advice had been sought from the Welfare Department. In a letter dated 31 July 1969, the Chairman of the Management Committee wrote to the Chief Welfare Officer, telling him of a possible new matron, who had the qualification of SRN, and indicating that his Committee would try to abide by the suggestions of the Welfare Department. However, it is clear from correspondence of 21 October 1969, that there had been no change of matron. And when the specialist Welfare Officer visited the Home on 9 December, he found that the new Matron had left after only one week, and that the old Matron had since returned to her post.

The residents

A major object of the visits to the Home by the specialist deaf Welfare Officer, was to report on and assess the residents for whom his own local authority was responsible, and to provide similar information to other local authorities which were responsible for other residents there. Indeed, so seriously did the Welfare Officer take his responsibilities in this respect that on 9 January 1969, he requested background information on all out-of-borough residents, so that when he visited them on behalf of their own local authorities he could conduct an informed interview and make a thorough assessment. In his report of 9 January 1969, the specialist Welfare Officer set the residents against the background of their 'austere and silent surroundings', and talked of their 'drabness of dress', and despite his best efforts to converse with them, concluded that, in fact, they had little to talk about because of their restricted lives. His skills in manual communication did not help him with two of the women, both of whom were deaf and blind, and thus themselves did not sign. Although the ages of residents ranged from the 20s to the 70s, most were elderly and had spent a considerable proportion of their lives at the Home. One deaf/blind resident had lived there for 50 years, while another had been there for 44 years and could remember the occasion on which the original Home had moved to the present building in 1932. It appears that, most unusually, the majority of residents had maintained close contact with relatives over the years. [1] On 15 July 1969, a visit to the Home disclosed that two of the deaf women for whom the borough was directly responsible had been ill. The odd defiant act by the residents was appreciated by visitors from the Department. The specialist Welfare Officer recorded in his account of his visit to the Home on 9 December 1969, that one of the ladies liked to smoke; this was against the rules; however, emboldened by his presence, she enjoyed a cigarette during her interview with him.

It is clear from the pressures which they applied to the Borough, that other local authorities with residents at the Home intended that monitoring and supervision of the establishment should be a reality: it is evident in a number of cases that a good deal more than a laissez faire relationship between Borough and voluntary Home was required. For example, on 3 February 1969, the Chief Welfare Officer of an Outer London Borough conveyed his thanks for a report on one of his residents. On 10 February, the Chief Welfare Officer reported to his counterpart in a West of England County on one of that County's residents at the Home. On 31 July, the Chief Welfare Officer was in correspondence again with the same County to tell the welfare authorities there that a car took the Home's residents to Church once a week, and to report the holiday address of the resident for whom the County was responsible, and thanks were duly received on 14 August from the County.

Activities of residents

By 1969, much of the Townsend argument concerning the desirability of maintaining outside contacts in an effort to promote normality and maintain the interest of residents of homes in ordinary outside life had been absorbed by those working in local authorities. Therefore, it is not surprising to find, in a Department apparently wedded to promotional welfare that strenuous efforts were made to ensure that residents of the Home both went out and received visitors. The progress of these efforts was noted in the registration reports, but the practical pressure on the Home for change in this direction was applied by the specialist Welfare Officer and the Chief Welfare Officer.

In his report on his visit of 9 January 1969, the specialist Welfare Officer noted that the residents enjoyed their Christmas shopping expedition to Oxford Street. Because of the origins of sign language, even today, the lives of many deaf people are church centred, and this is particularly true of the elderly. There appear to have been considerable difficulties involved in getting the deaf residents of the Home to church, and so they were provided with a monthly service in sign lanugage at the Home. Both residents and Welfare Officer regarded this arrangement as second best.

Going out was regarded as preferable to receiving services at Home, and by way of illustrating the point the Welfare Officer claimed to see an improvement in residents since they had begun to attend a club for the deaf. At this point he considered them to be happy 'despite their restricted life', and thought it essential that efforts should be made to ensure that they attended the new club which was about to be established by the local authority in a reorganisation of its day centre provisions. Within two months the arrangements for this change had been completed, though it is evident that in the process, messages had become garbled, wires crossed, and feelings hurt. On 3 March 1969, the Chairman of the Management Committee wrote to the Chief Welfare Officer expressing satisfaction regarding the new club, but explaining that residents could attend on only two days of the week as they had other things to do with their time, and reminding him of the importance of keeping Matron as well as the residents informed about the plans. On 19 March, the Chief Welfare Officer responded by writing to Matron to explain that there had been a misunderstanding - residents were to visit the new club on only one day a week. Special functions would be held for the deaf and the deaf/blind on Wednesday mornings between 10 a.m. and 12.45 p.m. Afterwards, lunch would be provided and residents would leave for home at 2 p.m. As there would be a transport problem, he hoped that some of the residents would be able to make their own way there and back. The same information was carefully conveyed to the Chairman of the Management Committee on the same day.

The new arrangements did not necessarily extend external contacts in the way expected. By the time the registration report was made on 15 July 1969, it was clear that although residents had been on a half day outing, shopping expeditions in the locality, and a holiday in Margate, they had not been on any outings since all the clubs had been moved to the new centre. However, those who were blind and deaf now attended a special club once a month, and there appeared to be a prospect that the Chaplain would be able to take some residents to Church once a month. Teething problems regarding attendance at the new centre continued, and on 21 October 1969, the Chief Welfare Officer wrote to Matron agreeing that the Wednesday outing to the centre did not appear to be a success, and that they should return to their Monday visits, though those who wished to do so could continue to go to craft on Wednesdays. Despite these efforts, the Registration Officer reported on 9 December 1969, that residents still missed their old club.

Even the annual Christmas shopping expedition was dependent upon intervention by the Welfare Department. On 31 October 1969, the Chief Welfare Officer wrote to Matron to report that he was now negotiating with the British Red Cross for arrangements to be made regarding the annual visit to the shops to be made before Christmas, which this year was to be paid to Woolworth in Oxford Street: did she wish her residents to be included?

In contrast to the effort put into ensuring that residents got out of the Home, there were few attempts to extend the range of people who visited the Home. An exception was the visit of fundraising walkers to the Home in 1969. However, there were others besides the employees of the Welfare Department, the chaplain, the doctor and the chiropodist who visited the Home. Among the volunteer visitors was an 87 years old woman who helped the residents with their needlework. And on at least one day that year, the Home opened its doors to the rest of the world: on 8 August an Open Day and Sale of Work took place, attended by the Mayor. No doubt the craft, which, apart from watching television was the main occupation of the residents, was appreciated not only by the Mayor but by its 87 years old supervisor.

The new matron

Considerably less interaction between the Home and the Local Authority is recorded for the following year. Presumably the routine which had been established in the previous year was running sufficiently smoothly for little intervention to be required. But there was another reason why the Department might have wished to hold back: 1970 saw the appointment of the new Matron. Perhaps both sides were feeling their way towards an acceptable accommodation; perhaps, too, the requirement to intervene appeared to be less urgent as the approach of the new Matron to her job emerged as being far more acceptable to the Department than had been true of that of her predecessor. The momentous event of the new appointment was recorded in a note dated 5 February 1970 which reported that there was some difficulty in sorting out the financial contributions of residents. The new Matron was trying to sort out the books, the former Matron was too ill to help, and the residents were too confused to do so. Apart from the subsequent letter from the Chief Welfare Officer to the Secretary of the Management Committee in which the financial contributions of residents were finally sorted out, and the routine exchange of letters between the Chief Welfare Officer and Matron regarding the arrangements for the pre-Christmas shopping expedition (British Home Stores and Woolworth this year), the main point of interest was the new registration.

On 5 May 1970, the Chief Welfare Officer wrote to the new Matron telling her of the necessity for a new registration. The report of the registration visit of 25 August 1970 was far more enthusiastic than those of the past. Both the fabric of the Home and its Matron had improved. Not only had new equipment been bought for the laundry, but the curtains were now up in the dining room! To improve appearances and ensure another visitor to the Home, a hairdresser was now calling to attend to the hair of residents once a month. The Registration Officer reported that the new Matron was trying to make the Home more comfortable, but that she suffered from understaffing. The extra work she had undertaken to make the improvements and the time which she spent with residents meant that she had no free time. Certainly, the new Matron's style of letter writing was more enthusiastic, engaging, and direct than that of her predecessor. Typical is her letter of 11 November 1970, when, thanking the Chief Welfare Officer for his help, she reported the acquisition of an assistant, and concluded that she was now 'hoping to go forward and certainly scrapping the past of this place'. It is clear that by the end of 1970, Matron and Department had established a cordial relationship.

Once the new Matron had settled in, interaction between the Department and the Home remained almost at the level which had been achieved in 1969. It is striking and indicative of the relationship which had been estabished, that as soon as the new Matron encountered a major difficulty, she turned to the Department for help. That difficulty concerned the residents' annual holiday. On 17 February 1971, Matron wrote to the specialist Welfare Officer to report that the hotel which they were accustomed to use for holidays was no longer available to them, and to ask for his help. The immediate response was for the Chief Welfare Officer to invite Matron to use the Borough's holiday hotel - an offer which was gratefully accepted on 11 March. Thereafter, there was a flurry of activity by the Department to organise the financial arrangements for the holiday. On 24 March 1971, the Chief Welfare Officer wrote to his counterparts in the local authorities which also had responsibilities for residents at the Home, telling them of the cost of the holiday and asking if they were prepared to meet those costs. In the ensuing weeks affirmative replies dribbled back to the Department, and in late April, the Chief Welfare Officer was able to write to Matron informing her that the relevant local authorities had agreed to finance the venture. As soon as the holiday was over, Matron wrote to the Chief Welfare Officer to thank him for making the arrangements: her deaf ladies had enjoyed themselves, but they had been ostracised by the hearing holiday-makers, who had been rude about the group of signers in their midst; fortunately her ladies could not hear this, and she felt that the tight-knit group dependent upon sign had probably engendered jealousy in the hearing, who had felt left out in the face of such cohesion.

The Matron's second year was not easy. It became clear in 1971 that the fabric of the building of the Home was deteriorating. The approach of the Department was to apply gentle pressure to ensure that the necessary work was carried out, and with the new Matron installed they were probably confident that no more was necessary - they were pushing at an open door. It is apparent from a letter of 11 March that Matron herself was aware of some of the deficiencies of the building. On that date she wrote to the Chief Welfare Officer explaining that she was taking advantage of the holiday which he was arranging for her residents, to get the building redecorated while they were away. But more serious shortcomings soon became apparent. On 31 March 1971, the GLC Architects Department wrote to the Chief Welfare Officer about the deficiencies of the fire precaution arrangements at the Home, and insisted that work should be carried out immediately. The Chief Welfare Officer wrote to convey the news to Matron. Her response was immediate, and by 26 April 1971, she was able to inform the Chief Welfare Officer that all but one of the items listed had been attended to, and the remaining work would be done 'when the decorators return'. Certainly, by the time the reinspection visit was carried out on 7 June 1971, the work appears to have been satisfactorily completed. The Registration Officer reported that the day rooms had been improved, and that Matron was hoping to extend the central heating system.

During the course of the year, it is possible to discern a subtle shift in the relationship between Home and Department. It seems clear that the new Matron regarded the Chief Welfare Officer and his subordinates as her allies, and as a consequence there was as much pressure from her on them, as there was from them on her to extend the range of activities available to the residents. In her letter to the specialist

Welfare Officer on 17 February 1971, she reported in passing, that she had taken some of the residents to evening classes. By 7 June, the Registration Officer was able to report after her reinspection visit, that residents were now being visited by a preacher from a deaf club: the new matron was 'doing wonders; she was keen for the residents to get out and chat'. In a letter to Matron on 30 June 1971, the Chief Welfare Officer outlined the arrangements made by the Department for residents' outside activities: an art class on Wednesdays; one attended a braille class on Tuesdays; and in all cases lunch was included in the arrangements.

The interest of the Department in the residents as individuals continued, but it was now augmented by that of the Matron. She was clearly aware of the technological changes which had taken place over the years in audiometric testing and amplification, and seems to have formed the opinion, almost certainly correctly, that the residents of the Home had never been in a position to take advantage of such developments. On 17 February 1971, she reported to the specialist Welfare Officer that she was taking the residents for hearing tests and that she would be 'very pleased if (she) got a few hearing and talking'. This enterprise appears to have aroused interest in the causes of deafness among residents, for soon afterwards the Chief Welfare Officer considered it important to convey to Matron the news that the specialist Welfare Officer had discovered that one resident had become deaf as a result of 'the bombing and mental deficiency' - information which drew the thanks of Matron. Pressure from other local authorities continued for information about their own residents.

By the second half of 1971, the Department was able to view the Home with cautious approval. On 28 September, another local authority wrote to enquire if the Home would be suitable for a woman, aged 21, who was deaf without speech and mentally handicapped. Two days later, the Chief Welfare Officer replied with a brief description of the Home: with places for 32 women, it currently accommodated 24, whose ages ranged from the twenties to the seventies; although beds were in dormitories, there were curtains around each bed; each resident had a chest of drawers, and they shared wardrobes; residents were encouraged to help with the daily household chores; efforts were made to ensure that they got out of the Home, but there were difficulties in finding escorts.

Conclusion

Thus the Borough established in 1965, chose not to maintain

links with the voluntary Home through an informal arrangement whereby councillors, their wives, or ex-mayors sat on the Management Committee. Nor did it aim to maintain a watching brief and seek to influence the direction of the Home by the more direct route of acquiring a seat on the Management Committee for the Chief Welfare Officer. Instead, the widely neglected mechanism of the registration process was used to cajole the far from progressive regime of the Home to adopt care practices which more clearly reflectd the ideals of good practice which were being developed at the time. Given the nature of the buildings involved, it was unrealistic to advocate privacy and the greater acceptance of personal belongings, two increasingly widely accepted criteria upon which the achievement of a 'home like' atmosphere was considered to depend. In the circumstances, therefore, it was appropriate for the Department to concentrate on the achievement of physical comfort through the upgrading of furnishings, especially in the provision of lampshades, curtains and carpets, and to encourage interaction between residents and local community outside the Home.

It is surprising that this promotional approach to welfare was directed so assiduously at a voluntary home, and even more unusual that a home for the deaf was chosen for all this attention. At a time when residential care was suffering from something of an eclipse as a desirable policy option, it was becoming fashionable to concentrate ideas for improvements in services on domiciliary and community provision. Furthermore, the low priority usually accorded to services for the deaf, because of the communication problem, and particularly to such services as they had which were traditionally the province of the voluntary organisations, as was unquestionably the case with residential accommodation, made the Home a particularly unlikely target of such attention. And the policy was only possible with the active engagement of a social worker for the deaf who possessed good skills in manual communication. In the circumstances, it seems clear that an interested Chief Welfare Officer, determined upon a policy of promotional welfare, decided that in the case of a voluntary Home for the deaf, such a policy could acquire meaning only through a combination of the deliberate and systematic use of registration and the establishment of a specialist post for the development of services for deaf people.

NOTES

[1] One of the major objections to residential care is the way it distances residents from their families. See Townsend, P., op. cit., and Sainsbury, S., Deaf Worlds.

6 The Home and the Borough 1972 to 1983

In 1972, important changes took place in the administrative structure of the personal social servicers, and it is the purpose of this chapter to assess the impact of these changes on the relationship between the Home and the Borough until 1983, when the Home experienced a crisis in its fortunes. It is important at the outset, however, to consider the changes in ideas about the personal social services which had taken place during the 1960s, for these determined not only the nature of the administrative changes which took place in the 1970s, but also the policies adopted for the different services. The Report of the Seebohm Committee will be the focus for discussion because this not only prompted the administrative changes, but also encapsulated many of the ideas which were to be such a formative influence on practice. Pressure for the Committee's proposals emanated from two main sources: first, there was the desire for the unification of the social work profession which had become a preoccupation among leading professionals, and particularly the leading social work teachers; and second, there was the requirement that something should be done about juvenile delinquency.

Pressures for service and professional unification

Even as long ago as 1959, it had been possible for Younghusband to argue that the basis for a single training and a single profession already existed in the rapid development of the social sciences which had taken place in the immediate past and which showed evidence of continuing; moreover, it was claimed that there was clear evidence for a single discernible social work task within the myriad activities which could be identified as having a social work element. [1] In the circumstances it seemed appropriate to deplore the lack of training of most of those identified as being engaged in some way in social work. Even the majority of child care officers were untrained, although their training courses were undersubscribed, and as a group they were, after psychiatric social workers, the most likely to be trained. And it was common to deplore as parochial the sectional specialisms which had grown up informally in relation to particular client groups, and which were typified by welfare department practice. Despite widespread acceptance of the Report's analysis, the Younghusband solution of a single profession divided into two tiers according to the difficulty of the task undertaken, not client group, failed to win acceptance.

However, it was in relation to services for children that the most important pressure for service and professional unification arose. Alarm was generated in the 1950s by a rising rate of juvenile crime, which was taking place despite the major social reforms of the early post-war years. It had been supposed that the abolition of want through a universal social security system and the guarantee of work through full employment, free universal education at secondary level, the availability to all of health care which was free at the point of provision, the programme of slum clearance and so on, would together abolish the main social problems which, it was thought, gave rise to crime. Government concern found expression in the establishment of the Ingleby Committee in 1956, [2] the first of a series of committees on the subject which were to sit and report in the 1960s. In the event, in many ways, the reaction to Ingleby proved to be more important than the Report itself. In its refusal to abandon the juvenile court, the Committee was regarded by progressives in the field of child care, both practitioners and academics, as hopelessly timid. In many ways such reaction was typified by the three Fabian Essays produced in response to the Report. Donnison's contribution, in particular, in its insistence on the importance of establishing common services and treatment for children in need and those convicted of crimes, and in its repetition of the Younghusband plea for improving coordination and cooperation between the different services involved with children by reducing their number through the creation of a family service, not only encapsulated the progressive position on the child care question, but also did much to strengthen the hand of those who sought the unification of the social work profession. [3] Two subsequent reports, that produced by Lord Longford's Committee [4] for the Labour Party while it was in opposition, and The Child, the Family and the Young Offender, produced in 1965, [5] essentially reiterated the Donnison position: there was no essential difference between children in need and those who had committed crimes; therefore, the juvenile court should be abandoned, and the two groups of children should be treated by the same set of services; and as it was imperative to establish cohesive services for children, the number of separate services involved should be reduced and replaced by a family service. Although it is true that the final report of the decade on the question - Children in Trouble [6] - retreated on the issue of the juvenile court, adherence to the notion of a single service for children through a family service was largely retained. It is important to note at this stage that the most influential voices calling for service unification were doing so from the perspective of the child care field.

However, although Donnison's starting point was the Ingelby Report and children's services, in the later stages of his essay he argued for the inclusion of other groups within his proposed family service, and the conscious adoption of a community or neighbourhood based approach for such services. Furthermore, the Ingleby Report, in proposing that a committee should be set up to enquire into the structure of the personal social services also furthered the cause, for the sequel to its proposal was the Seebohm Committee. Although it was initially set up to consider the structure of a family service, the Seebohm Committee, under influential pressure from outside government, succeeded in extending its terms of reference to include all clients of the personal social services. [7] The ensuing awkwardness of its position is illustrated by its failure to consider the needs of all clients within the context of a family service: to the contrary, these were discussed from the point of view of each of the separate client groups. The failure to deal effectively with the difficulty that many clients of personal social services did not live in families led the Committee to propose a single local authority service based on generic social work without offering guidelines as to how many elderly, mentally disordered, or disabled people were to be fitted into such a service. In a unified service, specialisms, too, became a problem. While it was admitted that the necessity for specialists would continue, it was unclear both how they would fit into a generic framework, and how they would be reproduced in the future, once the current specialisms acquired mainly through experience of working with a particular group of clients had disappeared through retirement or other causes from the social work arena. Indeed, there was little appreciation of groups in the Report: where specialisation was discussed, it was in the context of particular methods of work - community work and management and administration - for which it was suggested that there should be advanced courses in universities. [8] The main focus of the Report was on a single, generic service, and, therefore, it was not surprising that it was this which attracted most attention and which dominated the implementation of the Local Authority Social Services Act 1970, the statute by which the Report was given practical expression.

Genericism and specialisation

The new social services departments which were set up in the wake of the Social Services Act by the county and county boroughs and the metropolitan boroughs were forced to attempt to reconcile services organised generically with responsibilities outlined by statute according to client group. The response was ad hoc rather than based on any thorough assessment of how the problem should be overcome, but a general pattern emerged: the elderly were dealt with by untrained or assistant social workers, and the general classes of the physically handicapped by occupational therapists. Trained generic social workers tended to be reserved for children and families - the groups who originally had provided the springboard for the Seebohm reforms. With the widespread adoption of generic caseloads, the parochialism which had generated intense loyalty to a particular client group such as the blind or the deaf, disappeared, as did any focus for the championship of their special needs. As a consequence, specialist workers for the blind and deaf began to disappear, partly as a matter of policy, but partly through promotion, retirement, or movement out of local authority service. Although many blind people objected to what they considered to be a dilution of their services, the deaf generally had less to lose, were less able to voice their objections, and in any case, in many areas, their services had not been integrated into those directly provided by the local authority. Nor was there much opposition to such changes from social policy analysts and others who were interested in such groups. During the 1960s, it became fashionable to insist upon the similarities rather than the differences between the various categories of disabled people. Specialist services and specialist voluntary interest groups alike were condemned for parochialism, and the new approach was reflected not only in academic writing on disability, [9] but also in the establishment of new pressure groups representing the interests of all categories of disabled people. Indeed, symptomatic of the change was the increasingly widely adopted use of the generic term 'disabled' in the place of the myriad differentiating labels of the past. The new generic approach had much to do with the desire to rationalise the existing social security system, and ensure an adequate maintenance for members of all groups of disabled people, both men and women. The search for a disability income encouraged research and discussion to focus on the problems of counting disabled people, and therefore of defining and measuring disability.

Indeed, the growth of self-help campaigning groups among disabled people, which reflected the growth of participatory and consumerist ideas among welfare beneficiaries generally in the late 1960s, was both a reflection of, and in itself led to an increasing political awareness among such groups. To some, the welfare services appeared to be incapable of responding to any needs other than those of the professionals and administrators who organised and allocated them. As disability began to be seen in terms of choice and control, the passivity associated with the receipt of services appeared to become inappropriate: a disability income would enable those who required it to buy the help they needed on their own terms. However, although much campaigning effort and skill, as well as research time, was devoted to the achievement of a freedom-giving income, many continued to press for an extension of rights in terms of access - to public buildings, transport, and employment, and improved welfare services. The Chronically Sick and Disabled Persons Act 1970 appeared to many to meet such desires. But the slow progress noted by those monitoring the Act [10] diluted the faith of some in the capacity of the welfare authorities to respond satisfactorily, while the success in some quarters of the choice and control argument at a time when an adequate disability income appeared to be a political possibility, encouraged an ambivalent attitude towards services, and the professions by which they were promoted and dispensed. Thus some of the pressure which might have been brought to bear on local authorities to extend and improve their services for disabled people was diverted to other, more attractive objects. Nevertheless, pressure groups of disabled people or those operating on their behalf, were successful in ensuring a continuing, and, indeed, increasing rate of growth in services provided by local authorities for disabled people in the 1970s.

Residential care

However, residential care, the service with which the present study is concerned receded still further as a focus of policy attention. The Seebohm Report reflected a growing body of academic and pressure group opinion in adopting an increasingly fashionable concern for 'community'. For the Seebohm Committee, a major objective was a reciprocal arrangement between the new social services department and the local community in making provision for those groups for whom it was necessary. Residential care was widely castigated as expensive, for its failure to ensure for recipients a 'normal' way of life, and cost effectiveness in therapeutic terms. The revelations of Sans Everything, [11] and the Ely Hospital Report [12] not only aroused popular support for government policy to close the long-stay hospitals, but also added urgency to the process. As a consequence, attitudes which had previously reflected an ambivalence towards residential care, now hardened into outright hostility towards it. The discredit into which the long stay hospitals had fallen spilled over to affect all residential care. Although there were some experiments in extending the control of disabled people over the manner in which they lived in residential homes, these were isolated cases: the main objective was now to remove at least the young disabled and chronic sick - that is, those below retirement age - from such institutions. Little thought was given to the plight of older people in residential care, or to determining what good residential care would look like. Indeed, except, perhaps, for ideas about block treatment and so on elaborated by Tizard et al [13] in relation to mentally handicapped children, little advance was made during the 1960s and 1970s on the ideas of Townsend in this respect.

Thus, by 1972, specialisation which had developed informally through practice with particular groups of recipients of services provided under the National Assistance Act 1948, was under attack. The amalgamation of the local authority personal social services into a single social services department was undertaken largely in the interests of children and families, and in an attempt to deal more effectively with child offenders. Not surprisingly, professional generic social workers found their time increasingly engaged with these rather than the less politically sensitive groups. The trend was confirmed in 1974 when the Maria Colwell Report heralded the problem of child abuse as a dominating concern for local authority social services departments. As informal specialisms arising from experience disappeared through promotion, retirement and so on, disabled people became less and less likely not only to find help from welfare workers who understood their problems, but even from trained social workers. [14] And the response from disabled people themselves was muted partly by an increasing tendency to see themselves and to be seen by others as belonging to a generic category - the disabled. [15] In part, too, although pressure group activity was sufficient to maintain the necessity for an increasing level of welfare services for disabled people, it was diluted by the campaign for a disability income. Therefore, as a result of structural changes in the administration of services, disabled people found themselves pushed to the margins of concern in terms of the major preoccupations of the main professional group employed by social services departments, namely, social workers. And for those in residential care, especially if they were above retirement age, the increasing hostility to institutional provision in general, reinforced the development.

The Home 1972

The establishment of a social services department in place of the previous health, welfare, and children's departments, had no immediate and dramatic impact on the relationship between the Borough and the Home. No doubt this is to be explained in part by the retention of personnel who had been key figures in creating and promoting the existing relationship. The specialist Welfare Officer for the deaf continued to be employed by the new department throughout 1972. The Registration Officer remained in post. The Chief Welfare Officer became Associate Director Care Services, and it was he who continued to play a directional role in the relationship. However, the number of items in the records relating to that relationship, dropped dramatically compared with previous years, to only seven items in all. To some extent, the reduction in recorded interaction may have been due to the fact that expectations and satisfactory responses on both sides had been established. Certainly, correspondence in May 1972, between Department and Home, and with other departments involved in the financial arrangements for the residents' annual holiday, had acquired all the aspects of the routine for everyone involved. And the satisfaction of the Department with the approach of the new Matron at the Home is manifest in the Registration Report on the visit, dated 20 January: the 'marked improvement' which had taken place in the Home was emphasised by the Registration Officer. The report of the Specialist Worker on his visit to assess individual residents at the Home in May, commented on the success of the visit, and noted that all were well. Pressure continued for the continuation of this process of individual assessment from other local authorities who required information on their own residents at the Home. But it is evident that satisfaction with the Home was not considered to preclude new initiatives: the continuing interest on the part of both Matron and the Department in extending the range of opportunities for residents to acquire new interests and outside contacts is reflected in a May letter from Matron conveying her thanks for arrangements made for residents to attend an art class. The importance attached to such activities by everyone in the Home is made clear from Matron's observation that, as was the case with all such visits to clubs, residents 'can't wait to get there'.

That there was a continuation of the developing reliance by Matron on the Department in her attempts to improve the physical amenities of the Home, and that she tried to use the Department's support for this purpose against her own Management Committee is clear from the Registration Officer's report. Matron was in striking disagreement with the Committee on the type of expenditure which was being made: on the one hand she objected to the purchase of a deep freeze for the Home because she did not consider that the number of residents justified the initial expense or the running costs; on the other hand, flashing lights were still required yet she had been unable to persuade the Honorary Treasurer to transfer sufficient money from the investment to the current account to pay for such improvements. Indeed, Matron appears to have been left by the Management Committee to some extent to struggle on her own as best she could, and was described on the occasion of the registration visit as wrestling with the balance sheet. It was to the Department that she turned for aid with a request for help from the Borough auditor with the accounts. However, the Management Committee too, was becoming accustomed to seek aid and advice from the Department. By now, the age of the buildings of the Home and their unsuitability for accommodating an aging resident population was forcing the Management Committee to consider how best to meet the increasingly stringent modern safety requirements and the comfort of residents. In the event, it was agreed to seek finance for a fire escape, and a lift to enable elderly and impaired residents to move between the floors of the Home with greater ease. In May, the Director of Social Services asked the Borough finance officers if they could help with a loan towards the cost of these improvements: the £4000 to £6000 in question could not be raised by the Home whose voluntary funds were exhausted.

In June there was an intimation that more substantial changes were taking place in the structure and personnel of the Borough's Department of Social Services. In that month, a senior social worker, not the Associate Director, signed the letters regarding the annual holiday for residents.

The Home 1973

During 1973, there was no increase in contact between Department and Home: seven items were again recorded in the files. In many respects, the year emerges from the records as one of crucial change. Stability and continuity are represented by only one exchange between Matron and the Assistant Director: on 15 February, Matron wrote to thank the Department for arranging for residents of the Home to attend art classes, and she portrayed those who were to go as being in a state of high anticipation. But there was no mention that year of a specialist worker for the deaf, though a personal care officer was appointed. Moreover, the duty of registering the Home was undertaken by a new officer. In January, the new Inspector recorded her visit to the Home to introduce herself and report that all was well in a short handwritten note. When an Outer London Borough requested information regarding its own residents at the Home, it was the Inspector who prepared the reply on 14 May with a short handwritten report on the three people concerned and the Home. Even the annual holiday began to be queried. On 22 May, a county required further information regarding the resident for whom it was responsible as well as the holiday on the grounds that it was no longer the authority's practice to pay for holidays automatically for those in homes. The impression given by the records at this point is of the beginning of a narrowing of concern, at least for deaf people in residential accommodation at policy making levels in the new departments. And doubts about the future of the Home itself began to arise as it became clear that the fire escape and the lift, both of which were apparently beyond the income of the Home, were not the only items of major development required. On 13 July the problem of paying for rewiring the Home was raised, and the plan to meet the cost from the Borough's accumulated fund and to raise the fees charged to residents to repay the debt was devised and agreed. In August the fees were duly raised.

The Home 1974-77

The effect of the changes in personnel and structure which were a major feature of 1972 and 1973 and which culminated in 1974 in the appointment of a new Director had a marked and immediate effect on the relationship between the Home and the Borough in the following years. There are only two references in the records in each of the four years 1974 to 1977 to the Home. [16] Not only the number, but also the content of the communications concerning the Home contracted dramatically. During these years no registration visit was recorded. There is only one brief handwritten report concerned with the Home and the welfare of its residents, and that was prepared as a reply to a request from an outer London borough for information regarding one of its residents: on 12 June 1974, the Home was declared to be much improved and the resident concerned well. Thereafter, the question of individual welfare and the Home's regime cease to be concerns recorded in the file. Thus there are no references in these years to the activities of residents. It is impossible to learn from the records if the residents continued to go to church, attend their clubs and classes, enjoy their Christmas shopping expeditions and go on holiday. There is no evidence that the Department continued to pursue a policy of promotional welfare and active intervention. The few items of correspondence for these years are concerned mainly with matters of finance, and none of these were initiated from within the Department. Thus on 12 March 1974, a query was sent to the Personal Care Officer regarding the maintenance fees of one of the residents. But others concerned the financial difficulties of the Charity responsible for the Home, and related to attempts by the Charity to pressure the Borough into providing help. On 19 September 1975, the Chairman of the Management Committee explained to the Director of Social Services that because the large scale renovations required by the Home in recent years, such as the installation of a lift and rewiring, had created considerable financial difficulties for the Charity, they would have to increase their charges substantially or reduce their investment income by realising their assets, a course of action likely to produce long term problems. The Director's response on 20 October 1975, declared the innovations, such as the installation of the lift, to be reasonable in view of the increasing age of the residents. In the following year, on 1 June 1976, the Borough Accountant replied to the Management Committee's proposals: they should realise some of their investments, borrow the rest at market rates from the Borough, and recoup by charging higher fees. On 10 June 1976, the Chairman of the Management Committee was informed that the Borough had agreed to a loan of £12,500.

Only two other items appear in the records for these four years. One, which was relatively routine and insignificant, concerned the invitation to the Director to attend the Annual General Meeting of the Charity on 29 October 1977, an invitation which was declined. But the other was more significant - a note regarding the cancellation of the Registration Certificate of 5 May 1970, and the need for a new report.

It seems clear that from 1974 onwards, there was no desire to actively intervene in the running of the Home, to maintain and improve standards, either through the registration process, a specialist worker, or the interest of a Chief Officer. The triumvirate which had been crucial to the maintenance of a promotional policy with regard to the Home, had been destroyed. Registration visits were not systematically pursued, there was no longer a specialist worker, and the interested Chief Officer had disappeared. The Borough appeared to see its role merely in terms of reacting to requests for help and so on from the Home. By the mid-1970s, these were concerned almost entirely with problems relating to the fabric of the building, and the difficult financial consequences for the Charity of attempting to deal with them. It is in these years, when the welfare of residents ceased to be a direct concern of the Department, and policy had switched from one of intervention to one of reaction, that the Home emerged as being typical of those voluntary homes described by Townsend in the late 1950s - always in financial difficulties, always trying to make ends meet. However, by the mid-1970s, the problem was exacerbated by aging buildings which required substantial renovation, and accommodation which was becoming inappropriate for an aging community. The reaction of the Borough was to facilitate loans with little consideration of the deep underlying plight of the Charity. The problems of the Home were now of far greater moment than a question of lampshades or curtains, or even floor coverings, and in many ways resembled those faced by government with regard to the long stay hospitals. Old buildings, suffering from past lack of investment, could be adapted to modern standards of performance only with a large financial outlay: in the case of the hospitals government decided to abandon them altogether. Later evidence indicates that from 1974 onwards, the Department relied entirely on the local area office to maintain the relationship with, and give support to the Home. But there is no indication of concern as to how, or if this was being done, nor of any particular policy which was to be adopted towards the Home. The Home had ceased to exist as far as the Department was concerned - except when it demanded attention. An unspecific watching brief was devolved to an Area Office.

The search for a role: 1978

The year 1978 brought a striking contrast with the immediate past: there was a flurry of interaction between the Department and the Home which was at a level unequalled since 1971. To begin with, there was the first visit to the Home for registration purposes since 1972. It is clear from the records that this arose out of necessity for a new registration certificate rather than from a reintroduction by the Department of the systematic use of registration visits to monitor progress and influence the regime of the Home. The visit was undertaken by an Officer new to registration in terms of the Home's history, on 28 June 1978. A recent increase in the level of staffing was reported, but it was also noted that as the residents had become increasingly elderly and more dependent, an even higher level of staffing was required. The references to the residents themselves were oddly at variance with those of the recent past: the Registration Officer reported that as the residents were now elderly, and for the most part had lived at the Home for between 20 and 30 years, they resisted attempts to involve them in the outside world. There is no hint here of the eager anticipation with which residents were recorded as viewing the prospect of a shopping expedition, or attendance at an art class only four years previously. Perhaps the failure of an Officer new to the Home to acquire a signing companion for the visit ensured that the residents' views were not adequately explored and the implications of deafness not understood. Another possibility, of course, is that in the absence of direct pressure from the Borough, the Home's regime had regressed to the narrow and minimalist approach which had prevailed there before the interventionist policy of the Borough had begun to have an effect on care practice in 1969.

Apart from the Registration visit, the only move with regard to the Home initiated by the Borough concerned payments for residents attending the Day Centre. In the retrenchment following the publication of the Priorities Document in 1976, [17] retrenchment rather than promotional welfare was the main policy objective with regard to the Home. On 24 June 1978, the Director of Social Services wrote to colleagues in other social services departments with residents at the Home, to ask them to pay for those residents' attendance at the Centre. That the Borough was not alone in insisting on retrenchment even at this level is clear from one reply to the letter, to the effect that no such payment would be made unless assurance could be given that other local authorities were complying with the requerst; and if such a payment were to be made, would be Borough please deduct it from the maintenance fee accordingly? The Borough was able to give the assurance required but refused to lower the maintenance fee.

The problems of the building which housed the Home continued the preoccupy the Management Committee, and these worries were pressed on the attention of the Department and the Borough. It was made clear to the Department that the Home required new baths and plumbing, and a little later the Department was informed that the GLC required that the Home's fire prevention arrangements be upgraded. The Management Committee had put the work out to tender and the lowest they had received was for £9000. In view of the financial predicament of the Charity and the experience of the recent past, perhaps it is not surprising that the Management Committee's immediate response should be to ask the Borough for a loan of £10,000 - a request which was granted. It is striking that such a loan appears to have been made with no systematic assessment of the Home, its role and finance, nor any attempts to exert an influence over a facility to which a loan committment was made. Withdrawal from a policy of promotional welfare may be understandable, given that such a policy was not common in the context of voluntary residential provision, especially for the deaf, and retrenchment may be regarded as acceptable following the cuts in the growth of social services inaugurated by government in 1976. What was odd was the willingness to make a loan to a charity without thorough investigation as to its objectives and practices. When such concerns were raised as issues, it was not by the Borough but by the Management Committee.

In June 1978, arrangements were made at the request of the Chairman of the Management Committee for a meeting with the Director of Social Services to consider the future role of the Home. The prospect of lunch with the Chairman, the occasion favoured by the Management Committee for the discussion, did not find favour with the Director. On 6 June, the Director's note regarding the arrangements suggested the desirability of a change of plan: 'The only embarrassment about this is that I was invitd to lunch - a party of three is rather heavy. Could you please ring - and confirm date, but ask if he would prefer us to come after lunch.' The outcome of the meeting was the decision that the Director should circulate fellow directors in the Greater London area with details of the Home and its objectives, asking them to give some indication of the use they expected to make of such a facility in the future. It is a measure of the distance which had developed between the Home and the Borough since 1972, that on 12 July 1978, in commenting on the letter sent out on 4 July to other social services departments, the Chairman of the Management Committee, while agreeing the general text, found it necessary to point out that the number of residents at the Home was 19, not 21 as the letter had suggested, and reported that Matron had been consulted on the matter of the letter generally.

Within a little more than a week, replies to the letter began to be received by the Director, and by the end of August most of the local authorities contacted had replied. The replies are of interest for the evidence they provide that deaf specialist workers were once more beginning to be appointed by local authorities. [18] In fact, it may be the case that in some areas there had been no discontinuity between the practice of the welfare department and that of the social services department in this respect. The replies from the three local authorities with specialist appointments are striking for their length and the fact that some systematic thought had been given to the problem posed: in each case the director's reply was based on a report from the deaf specialist worker. The relative brevity of the replies from departments with no such specialist is illustrated by one borough, whose director reported on 15 August 1978, that they employed no specialist worker directly, though they used the services of RADD, and they had no suggestions to make regarding the Home. Another director who employed no specialist wrote on 17 August to explain that while they had Blind/Deaf people, who required residential care, they were likely to be catered for in a local home for the blind since this was regarded as their main disability.

A further striking feature of the replies is the evidence they give of the widespread unpopularity of residential care facilities of the traditional type. One borough replied on 4 September, that a 'community' response was preferred for younger people, though it was conceded that residential care would be required in the future for elderly deaf people, especially for short stay relief, though self-contained flats were the most desirable solution for meeting the needs of non-dependent older deaf women. Another director saw a demand for short term residential supportive care for the younger deaf who were experiencing difficulties living in the community. Yet another possibility suggested was for a home for the elderly deaf or one for younger people designed to prepare them to deal with the difficulties of working and running a home as independent adults. It was the policy of another local authority to integrate the elderly deaf into homes for the hearing elderly.

All of these replies were made by directors unaided by the presence of a specialist worker, and it seems clear that in coming to their conclusions they were extrapolating from the accepted wisdom regarding the use of residential care and applying it to the case of the deaf. It can be seen that traditional residential care was usually regarded as tolerable only for the dependent elderly and as a means of offering relief to caring relatives: in the case of younger people, to be acceptable, it had to be short stay and therapeutic. Most directors considered the fact that the Home catered for girls and women to be a difficulty: there was clear embarrassment at the thought of younger people and the elderly mixing within a single institution. Perhaps this objection was in some way connected with the campaign to remove the young chronic sick from long stay geriatric wards which had been generated by guilt at the discovery that such places were all that a tiny number of younger very dependent people could call home. Certainly, from the sociological point of view, it is difficult to understand objections to a residential home made on the grounds that it catered for a wide age range. After all, one of Townsend's major objections to homes for the elderly was that they segregated the generations. In these terms at least, a home for women and girls must be regarded as more normal than either a home for girls or for the elderly. More understandable in the sociological context was the objection raised by one director to a home catering for only one sex.

A few directors were puzzled by the combination of training and accommodation embodied in the Home's objectives. For training purposes a 'community' response was preferred to the residential: one director reported the use of the local further education college to train deaf youngsters as the appropriate model for effective training.

So far, only those replies from departments of social service where there were no specialist workers for the deaf have been discussed. It is interesting to consider, given the emphasis placed earlier on the importance of the specialist worker, whether directorial replies differed in any way other than length, when a deaf specialist was employed in a department. Perhaps the most obvious difference is the way in which knowledge of the deaf world and its services outside the range of local authority provision, is made apparent. Thus, on the basis of the deaf specialist's report, one director replied that the name of the Charity should be changed by replacing the words from 'Deaf and Dumb' with 'Prelingually Profoundly Deaf'; that as the only other home for elderly deaf women in London was full, it was important to maintain the accommodation provided by the Home; that the objectives of training and accommodation should be separated, and training programmes be devised in conjunction with the City Literary Institute, where there was a department specialising in the problems of deafness; and that training in household management, for which there was a real need among younger deaf people, would be best organised locally in the deaf clubs.

Another director had learnt from his specialist worker that it was now the policy of RNID to close its homes for the deaf: however, a hostel for young girls was required, as was a short stay specialist home for the elderly, and a half-way psychiatric facility. In this case, the viewpoint of RNID, that the elderly deaf should be moved from the specialist homes to residential care for the elderly run by local authorities, in the name of integration, was accepted without question. Specialist residential care was acceptable only for small clearly defined groups, and only if there was a therapeutic objective.

Thus, knowledge of the deaf world did not necessarily imply any real understanding of the problems associated with deafness. In such circumstances responses were as apt to reflect attitudes generally prevalent in the social services field and applied with little thought to the deaf, as were those in cases where no deaf specialist existed. But this was true of only one of the three departments where there was a deaf specialist on hand to advise the director. In the third case, the deaf specialist went so far as to spell out his objections to the RNID's policy: if, as RNID now required, elderly deaf people were put into homes for the elderly, they would experience such acute problems of communication that the standard of their care, as well as their mental health and general well being, would be profoundly and distressingly affected. He saw the Home's future as a regional resource which would include an assessment centre for deaf teenagers, and a training centre of maladjusted deaf girls.

On 6 October 1978, the Borough's Director of Social Services was able to write to the Chairman of the Management Committee that there were six departments in addition to that of the Borough among those contacted in London, 'who would like to be included in a future working party for consultation on planning and developments in the Home'. Two members of the Department, one of whom had signed the recent registration certificate, were identified as being suitable for inclusion in future discussions, and, the Director added, 'I will be happy to be of any further help personally if my advice would be helpful.' Attached to the letter were brief notes of the suggestions for the future development of the Home made by six of the boroughs from which replies to the original letter had been received. In essence, the ball had been thrown back into the court of the Management Committee. The Borough had reacted to a request from the Home, and the initiative was now once more with the Home. On the day that the letter was written to the Management Committee, the Director distilled for a fellow director, what was considered to be the essence of the replies of the London boroughs into the proposal that the Home should become a short stay educational centre for profoundly deaf women and girls. There are no other references in the records to this potentially important exercise. The members of the Management Committee were simply left to ponder its results.

Inactivity

In the following year, the records contain only three items of correspondence, all of which relate to the same topic. Once more, the initiative came from the Home. On 11 June, 1979, Matron wrote to the Department to convey her worry at the number of times the visits of the residents to the Day Centre had been cancelled in the previous six weeks: this had caused unhappiness because residents had got ready to go out, and had sat about in their outdoor clothes waiting in vain for the transport to arrive. On 18 June, a reply from the Department queried the number of times the problem had arisen, and blamed the incidents on lack of transport: when there was not enough space in vehicles to take everyone who required transport to the Day Centre, it was policy to leave the residents of the Home because they were in a setting where care was already guaranteed. On 28 June the Officer in Charge of the Day Centre wrote to Matron with the news that two more vehicles had been acquired; it was hoped, therefore that the transport problem had been overcome. This correspondence is of interest not only because it illustrates the marked change in the tone of the relationship between Home and Borough which had taken place since 1972, but also because it casts doubt on the Registration Officer's opinion of the previous year that the residents were unwilling to go out and mix socially with others.

The records are empty for the years 1980 and 1981. In March 1982, there is an item of correspondence relating to the cost of holidays. Silence descends once more in 1983. It is clear by this time that the Borough had allowed its relationship with the Home to deteriorate to a point at which it became vestigial, reactivated from time to time at the insistence of the Home's Management Committee. First, direct interest in the day to day regime of the Home and the welfare of its residents had been abandoned. Then, despite accumulating evidence of the shaky financial position of the Charity, the Borough appeared to be willing to shore it up by granting loans without displaying enough interest to investigate the situation. Finally, by failing to follow through the discussion on the future viability of the Home, which it had inaugurated at the insistence of the Management Committee, the Borough appeared to relinquish interest in even the very existence of the Home.

Given the history of the relationship between the Borough and the Home, an extraordinary situation had developed. The Borough was prepared to finance from its own public funds loans to the Charity without any thorough examination of the financial position of that body: no more was required than the presentation of the Management Committee's own perception of that position. Still less was there any assessment of the Home to determine whether it was an appropriate object of such help. When it was clear that in the eyes of the Management Committee the Home did not have a viable future, the Borough was able to inaugurate a London-wide discussion of possible alternative roles, report back to the Management Committee, and do no more, other than to express general interest and good will. There was no willingness to seek to ensure the well-being and future of its own residents or those of other boroughs at the Home for which it was the registering authority. There was not even an attempt to ensure that the object of its loans survived. Thus little obligation was felt by a public body to ensure that a voluntary organisation, dependent upon loans and maintenance fees from public funds, pursued an acceptable policy. Despite the considerable outlay of public funds through loans and maintenance fees, complete devolution to the Home had been achieved.

NOTES

[1] Younghusband, E., Report of the Working Party on Social Workers in the Local Authority Health and Welfare Services, London, HMSO, 1959.

[2] Report of the Committee on Children and Young Persons, London, HMSO, Cmnd. 1191, 1960.

[3] Donnison, D., Jay, P., Stewart, M., The Ingleby Report: Three Critical Essays, Fabian Research Series 231, 1962.

[4] Longford, Crime - A Challenge to Us All, 1964.

[5] Home Office, The Child, the Family and the Young Offender, London, HMSO, Cmnd. 2742, 1965.

[6] Home Office, Children in Trouble, London, HMSO, Cmnd. 3601, 1968.

[7] For a discussion on the establishment of the Seebohm Committee, see Cooper, J., The Creation of the British Personal Social Services 1962-74, Heinemann, 1983; and Hall, P., Reforming the Welfare: the politics of change in the personal social services, Heinemann, 1976.

[8] Report of the Committee on Local Authority and Allied Personal Social Services, London, HMSO, Cmnd. 3703, 1969.

[9] Sainsbury, S., Measuring Disability.

[10] Social Policy Research, The Implementation of the Chronically Sick and Disabled Persons Act 1970, Social Policy Research Ltd., 1973; Topliss, E., and Gould, B., A Charter for the Disabled, Basil Blackwell and Martin Robertson, 1981.

[11] King, R., Raynes, N., and Tizard, J., Patterns of Residential Care, Routledge and Kegan Paul, 1971.

[12] Keeble, U., Aids and Adaptations, Occasional Papers on Social Administration, Bedford Square Press, 1979.

[13] For a discussion of attempts to create a set of criteria by which the generic term disablement might be defined and disability assessed, see Duckworth, D., The Classification and Measurement of Disablement, DHSS, Research Report No. 10, HMSO, 1983.

[14] For a visual impression of the changes which took place at this point in the relationship between Borough and Home, see Appendix.

[15] DHSS, Priorities in Health and Personal Social Services in England, London, HMSO, 1976.

[16] By the late 1970s, the return of specialisation had begun to pose organisational problems for teams of social workers operating according to generic principles. See, Stevenson, O., Specialisation and Social Service Teams, George Allen and Unwin, 1981.

7 The Home and the Borough 1984 to 1986

In 1984, the Borough was forced to reconsider its policy of devolution and attempt to reassert a promotional relationship with the Home. It is significant that this did not occur as a result of a systematic and thorough examination of the Department of Social Services' administrative structure and policies, but from external pressures. The sources of these pressures were threefold. The first arose from changes in the government's social policy, and in particular its attitude towards and financing of voluntary and, more importantly, private residential homes. The release of public funds for maintenance fees to encourage the voluntary and private sectors to meet the growing demand for residential care had two immediate results. [1] The first was a rapid rise both in the number of private homes and in the levels of maintenance fees as owners of homes took advantage of the public largess. And the second was the growing clamour of objection as huge amounts of public money were seen to be handed over with no guarantee as to its appropriate use. The clamour was particularly shrill because the policy was initiated at a time when central government was substantially strengthening its control over local authority spending: the contrast in treatment was stark. To the first problem, the government responded by imposing an upper limit on the amount per head by which it would underwrite maintenance fees in residential homes. [2] The response to the second was the introduction of the Registered Homes Act 1984, which strengthened the control of registering authorities over residential accommodation in the voluntary and private sectors by requiring that every home must be registered by the Council and visited at least once every twelve months. Furthermore, a manual of good practice was to be made available to provide guidelines for assessment. [3] The Act was to prove to be the catalyst in the changing relationship between the Home and the Borough in the years 1984 to 1986.

However, without the intervention of a second factor, namely pressure from local voluntary groups acting on behalf of elderly and disabled people, it is possible that the Borough would not have pursued so vigorously the fate of the Home after the Registration Inspection visit. It could well have been the case that the Borough's interest would have been restricted to the formal application of the Act and the requirement that the health, safety and management standards were met, thus stopping short of any consideration of the long term consequences for the residents. One of the striking developments of the late 1960s and early 1970s was the degree to which participatory and pressure group politics by and on behalf of recipients and potential recipients of local services, and consumerism among the beneficiaries of such services, were successfully encouraged by social workers and others interested in countering the rigidities of the welfare bureaucracies, in some cases, with the hope of effecting substantial political change. [4] In the later 1970s and 1980s, such activities were increasingly regarded as an essential ingredient of local community politics, especially in inner city areas, especially by political parties which were left of centre. The two groups which were most active in the Borough with regard to the Home and its fate, showed energy, commitment, and an ability to use effectively the local media, including informal community news sheets, the formal local press, and local television.

The third factor to be taken into account when considering the reassertion of a promotional relationship between Borough and Home was the pressure exerted on the Social Services Department by those running the Home itself. By 1984, the predicament of the Home was thought to be so grave that those in charge of it were prepared to insist on a response from the Borough.

It is true that by 1985, the cause of services for the deaf was enormously strengthened by the appointment of two deaf specialists - a senior social worker and a social worker. Such appointments were indicative of a reappraisal of the need for specialisation in social services and a reflection of an increasingly widespread acceptance of specialist services throughout the London area, where most boroughs had already introduced specialist social workers for the deaf. However, in the case of voluntary residential services for the deaf it seems unlikely that the new specialist team was in a position to take the lead in the reappraisal of the relationship between the Home and the Borough. With time, aided by the Registered Homes Act 1984, and a Department determined to use that Act effectively to maintain standards, the role of the specialist worker in the Borough's old Welfare Department could have been replicated. But in the history of the Home and the Borough, the appointments came too late for such a development to take place.

Crisis - summer and autumn 1984

A measure of the urgency of the situation which became manifest in the second half of 1984 is that the records contain more items for the following two years than for the previous 15 years. Yet until August 1984, it appeared to be likely that the pattern of the previous decade was to be maintained: until then, there was only one item in the records for that year. In April, a request was received from the Charity's accountants that as from April 1 1984, the maintenance rate for residents of the Home should be raised from £50.61 to £96.29. The loan which had been granted by the Borough in 1978 had been paid off by the Management Committee in 1983. The rise in maintenance fees was required to pay for improvements to the fabric and staffing levels at the Home. It is a measure of the relationship between Home and Borough, which had remained unchanged for a decade, that the new rate was agreed to without investigation.

Yet, in fact, the Home and its Management Committee were in turmoil. Referring retrospectively to the events of the late summer of 1984, the then Acting Director of the Home informed the Director of Social Services on 8 December 1984, that at the August meeting of the Committee it became clear that the magnitude of the difficulties facing them were such that the Committee were united in the following resolution, namely, their inability to carry on running the Home.

> It was therefore resolved to take measures to close the house and arrange for the placement of its residents and the disposal of its residents and property. As a first step it was decided to make a request to the Director of Social Services of the Borough as to the best procedures to adopt.

It is striking that this information appears to have taken more than three months to reach the Borough's directorate, and arrived after the registration visit. On 30 October 1984, the Acting Director of the Home wrote to the Charity Commissioners informing them that the present Committee was unable to run the Charity as it was constituted, and that a Committee that could do so was required. In their reply of 14 November 1984, the Commissioners told the Acting Director that if the present trustees were unable to manage, others should be found. By 8 December, according to the Acting Director's letter, the Committee had transferred its responsibilities to a new Board, though the Registering Officer's report on the Home dated 31 January 1985, makes it clear that 'the present Committee of Trustees were not constitutionally elected'. Indeed the legality of the Committee of Trustees was to persist as a problem. Despite the resignation of some of the Board and the election of a new Executive Committee - unanimously, according to the minutes of the Extraordinary Meeting held on 9 February 1985, at a meeting with representatives of the Department of Social Services to discuss the Home's problems three days later, the Chairman of the Board confessed that he remained unsure of the legality of the new Committee. Nevertheless, he was encouraged on that occasion to act as the Home's representative by the Director of Social Services, and thereafter there appeared to be no doubt about his and his Committee's legal position.

As well as requiring advice from the Director, there was clear evidence from the Management Committee of a less formal but continuing relationship with the Borough. Indeed, the kind of relationship between voluntary home and local authority, whereby wives of councillors, ex-mayors, or senior members of the welfare department sat on management committees, which had been described by Townsend as occurring in the late 1950s, now emerged for the first time in the case of the Home and the Borough. But it is important to note that the development took place not as part of the Borough's determination to strengthen its relationship with, and therefore, its influence over the Home, but at the request of the Home's Management Committee which was in need of specific skills thought likely to be in evidence among the employees of the social services department, and perhaps, elected members. In a letter from the Charity Commissioners, to whom the members of the Management Committee had disclosed its difficulties, the Committee was urged, on 14 November 1984, to seek cooptions from the local authority.

Thus, in his letter of 8 December 1984, following the Registration Visit, the Acting Director of the Home told the

Director of Social Services that the new Board of Trustees should include people from the Borough's Social Services Department: his own term of office would end within the month, and in that event, the professional skills of the Department's officers and the support of the local councillors would be important. In fact, the arrangement which emerged was so informal that no one in the local authority was made officially aware of it, and in the case of one officer of the Authority, there remained ambiguity as to whether or not she was a member of the Committee. In a retrospective letter of 5 September 1985, the Assistant Director responsible for the Home, sought to explain the situation to an elected member: an officer of the Research and Planning Unit, in fact, had been coopted onto the Management Committee of the Home as long ago as 1983; thereafter, three other members of staff - the Home Management Officer (Day Care) and the head of the Day Centre which residents of the Home had attended for many years, had been asked to join the Committee by existing members because of the value attached to their knowledge of disability and committee procedures. They were all elected full members at the Extra Meeting held on 9 February 1985, and the Research and Planning Unit's Officer became the Management Committee's secretary in 1985.

Throughout 1985, there was some doubt about the status of the Personal Care Officer for the Elderly, who was also the Registering Officer for the Home, as well as being the wife of the new Chairman of the Management Committee. Although she appeared to have been elected to the Committee at the Extra Meeting of 9 February 1985, she was stated by the Assistant Director Care Services on 5 September 1985, when a question of a clash of interest had arisen, never to have been on the Management Committee of Trustees. Yet, in a handwritten note dated 5 November 1985, the Registering Officer was described as having met an officer of the local authority within whose boundaries new premises for the Home had been purchased 'in her capacity as a member of the Management Committee to discuss the move which was to take place tomorrow'. However, according to the minutes of the meeting of the Panel of Inquiry held on 21 November 1985, the Senior Social Worker for the Deaf reported that when he visited the new Home, he found this Officer running it, though, 'she made it plain that she was not a Trustee'. In contrast, the Assistant Director, at the same meeting explained that he had telephoned the new registering authority and had discovered that the Officer in question had visited that authority 'in the capacity of Registration Adviser for the Home, and presented herself as a Trustee'.

It seems clear from the records that the Borough's

Department of Social Services had neither sought as a matter of policy to strengthen its relationship with the Home by encouraging the cooption of suitable employees onto the Management Committee, nor responded to the suggestion from the Acting Director of the Home on 8 December 1984 that such cooptions would be welcome. As a result members of the Management Committee themselves were forced to search for contacts within the Department informally, presumably aided by the advice of the Departmental employee who was already a coopted member. In the event, therefore, those approached responded as individuals, and not as part, and, indeed, did not see themselves as part, of a mechanism through which Departmental influence could be brought to bear on the Home and its Management Committee. Indeed, so informal was the arrangement, and so divorced from the Borough's policy preoccupations, that those coopted did not feel any obligation to make an official disclosure of their position to their employers. The situation was to have unfortunate consequences for the residents of the Home, and to be the cause of considerable embarrassment to the Borough.

A major issue in precipitating the request by the Management Committee for help to the Department of Social Services was the question of the day to day management of the Home. Some time before June 1984, it appears that the Management Committee were so alarmed at the situation that they sought the help of a large voluntary association for the deaf and were provided with an adviser. However, the difficulties increased, and it appears from the Registration Visit Report of 31 January 1985, that in June 1984, Matron was dismissed, and the adviser became Acting Director. In responding to the Registration Visit in a letter to the Director of Social Services on 8 December 1984, the Acting Director described graphically the dimensions of the Home's difficulties: he had formerly been an adviser but was now directly involved in the Home as Acting Director because the situation had deteriorated to the point at which the Management Committee wished to close down the Home; the records and the office were in disarray; there was no effective management or day to day control; the staff had neither qualifications nor experience in the area; and there was barely legal coverage at night. The Acting Director's term of office was due to end on 31 December, and on 8 December, they still had no one to take over. The immediate crisis was resolved, however, by the appointment in January 1985 of a temporary acting person in charge. It was not until 21 June 1985, in his Report for 1984-5 that the Chairman of the Management Committee was able to announce that a woman, who, with her husband, had previously done voluntary work in the Home, had been offered the permanent post of Care Manager.

Indeed, so deep was the crisis perceived to be that in August 1984, the Acting Director conveyed the wish of the Management Committee to close the Home and the Charity to the Charity Commissioners. In the view of the Commissioners, however, the Trustees could take no such action if the Charity was viable, and beneficiaries were still in existence (14 November 1984). The contrast between the attitude of the Management Committee and that of the Social Services Department to the Home was sharp. The situation which had aroused such alarm in the Management Committee was viewed with equanimity by the Department. Explaining the Department's policy towards the Home retrospectively in an internal memorandum dated 15 October 1985, the Assistant Director reported:

> The Department of Social Services has always maintained contact with the Home through the local area Social Services office and as far as the Department is concerned, the interests of the three Borough residents and those of other local authorities were protected, and the standard of care considered to be satisfactory. As a consequence the standards employed by the Home have never been an issue for the Department.

Small wonder, then, that the Department failed to respond to the Management Committee's urgent request for cooptions. The policy of ignoring the possibility of using registration as a mechanism for control, or at least influence, and instead, devolving responsibility to an Area Office was never questioned. If the Area Office found no occasion for objections to the care practices at the Home - and apparently it never did - the Directorate was content to assume that there was no cause for concern. There is one item in the records of the Home which provides the substance of the case to support the sanguine view apparently taken by the Area Office. The picture which emerges is one which was made familiar in the Registration Reports of 1969 to 1972. It depicts the two Georgian houses knocked into one, standing in substantial grounds, and the, by now, mainly elderly residents; the six bedded rooms, the communal lounges, and large dining room. But a positive view was taken of many of the features of the Home which were to be interpreted negatively in the Registration Report of 1985. The fact that there were only three full time staff was regarded as providing the opportunity for the day to day running of the Home to be undertaken by the residents, even the frail managing to do something, so that they all benefitted from the feeling of being helpful. Although the care provided was admitted to be 'old fashioned', it was considered to be of a good standard. The Home was clean and tidy, the food simple but good. The staff were matriarchal but dedicated. A local GP visited regularly, and teachers went to the Home on four days a week to instruct residents in handicrafts. The residents went out regularly to the local Day Centre. And they enjoyed an annual holiday at Hayling Island. They attended a church service every Sunday taken by a local clergyman in sign language. The report concluded:

> A strange little community, somehow untouched by time, which provides good care, which is hard to see being provided by any alternative institution. In view of the age of the residents and the years they have been at the Home, this is the only place they can be.

Although the report is dated 12 March 1981, it was incorporated into the papers for the year 1985 in the records, perhaps with the intention of providing an antidote to the pessimistic attitudes towards the Home which were by then prevalent and to lend support to the Departmental view which had prevailed until the end of 1984. It seems certain that some deterioration had taken place since that date in the Home and its care regime, but this may have happened too quickly for the generic Area Office team to appreciate what had occurred, or it may be that the changes were not considered by social workers to affect materially the lives of residents. In addition, however, it is also clear that the situation in the Home was open to a variety of interpretations. Whatever the explanation, the Registering Officer's conclusions were markedly different from those of the Area Office social workers.

The question of registration

The visit to the Home by the Registering Officer took place on 27 November 1984. On 7 December 1984, she reported to the Director of Social Services: 'I visited this Home recently to inspect for registration under DHSS Registered Homes Act 1984 ... In my opinion and that of its Acting Director ... this Home falls far below acceptable standards in many important areas.' In her view deregistration was a matter requiring urgent discussion. In his response to the outcome of the visit, the Acting Director of the Home reinforced the opinion of the Registering Officer in a letter on 8 December 1984 to the Director of Social Services, by describing the needs of the Home as being 'desperate and urgent': although the residents could now move freely about the house, the lift which had been installed relatively recently did not serve all floors and only the more able residents could use it; there was no light call apparatus; there were wooden stairways and bare concrete steps. Four days later, the Registering Officer wrote again to the Director of Social Services, and referring to the question of the Home's deregistration, urged that the Home's situation was serious and that it was likely that a 'Prohibition notice under the terms of the Health and Safety at Work Act 1976' would close it.

It was not until the end of January 1985 that a full report on the registration visit was completed and the grounds on which the deregistration of the Home was to take place were fully documented. Taken as a whole, the catelogue of shortcomings is, without question, horrifying, and is an indictment of the the Borough's decade of non-intervention, and highlights the danger of devolving responsibility for the maintenance of standards to local units. It seems clear that the Area Office had grown used to declining standards. But this particular exercise in registration also points to some of the disadvantages of applying standard criteria without reference to particular histories, the general context of provision in particular fields, and the special needs of individual small groups. The defective fire alarm and escape system, the fact that the electric wiring was a hazard, that the kitchen and its equipment were unhygenic (the environmental health officials had visited in the recent past regarding an outbreak of illness among residents which was thought to be associated with contaminated food), that most of the building was without cold running water because of deficiencies in the old lead and iron plumbing system, was scandalous, but all of this could be rectified. The fact that some rooms, corridors and the main staircase were uncarpeted, and that the polished wood was a hazard, were minor difficulties which could be overcome easily, in the sense that they were not associated with the structure of the building. All that was required was the expenditure of funds.

However, other deficiencies were not of the same order, and offer proof that whereas it is easy to apply standard criteria with regard to fire, hygiene and so on, elsewhere, within limits, there is a place for judgement. The absence of adequate records for inspection was of importance though not necessarily of any great moment for residents. The conclusion that the 'tenuous' nature of the management structure gave rise to doubts about the ability to provide proper continuous care for residents is surely questionable: management problems need not be long term, and as we have seen, a short term solution was found after the departure of the Acting Director. Indeed, an Acting Person in Charge was already in post when the Registration Report was written, and thereafter a more permanent appointment was made. The doubts expressed regarding the quantity of other staff, and the quality of agency staff in particular with whom residents found it impossible to communicate, may be applied to most homes for the deaf. Recent research suggests that it is common for those running homes for the deaf to consider that their establishments are understaffed. Furthermore, it is regrettable that in most homes, only the person-in-charge is likely to be able to communicate in sign with residents, and then usually only at a rudiamentary level: residents tend to create among themselves close-knit communities, and interact very little with the hearing who run the establishments. [5] Again, this Home was not alone among residential estabishments for the deaf in the fact that 'the sleeping arrangements afford little privacy or any opportunity to maintain the quality of life.' [6] While in general, the use of even small dormitories must be condemned, in this particular case, their effect was not entirely negative. For this interdependent small community, which had been sleeping in these six bedded rooms for as long as 30 to 40 years in some cases, shared bedrooms were an advantage, as residents were able to help each other dress and undress more easily. However, it is not clear that similar advantages attached to the lack of privacy afforded by the 'washing and toilet facilities', though presumably the low quality fitments could have been replaced.

That change at the Home was possible, and, indeed, had already taken place, was admitted. Thus, in a letter to the Director of Social Services on 8 December, regarding the Registration Visit, the Acting Director reported that residents were now able to move about the building freely. And the Registration Officer's Report acknowledged 'the efforts of the Acting Director and the present Acting Person in Charge to improve standards and quality of life and care of the residents. Many areas are now considerably improved, particularly in respect of residents' needs as individuals and in the recent investigated records of the distribution of pocket money. Proper accounting is now being undertaken by a local firm of chartered accountants.' The reference to pocket money suggests that the Home's Matron had been indulging in a pratice common among heads of residential establishments - that of not only taking charge of pension books, but even withholding the statutory pocket money, which had been intended to guarantee that no one who sought shelter in residential accommodation would be rendered destitute as a consequence. In the interest of administrative convenience, it has become usual for the Person-in-Charge to hold pension books and dole out pocket money, but the tradition has grown up that they also exercise discretion in the distribution of pocket money, and in many cases refuse to hand it over, often on the flimsiest of excuses. Where this happens pocket money is usually forcibly saved or put into the establishment's comfort fund, but the practice itself, though widespread, is open to question, and the money involved may be subject to misappropriation. [7]

Despite the fact that changes had already taken place and most of the Home's difficulties could have been overcome with the expenditure of funds, and despite the fact, too, that the Home shared many characteristics with other homes for the deaf, as far as the Registration Officer was concerned, the only option open to the Social Services Department was to invoke its 'statutory duty and cancel the registration of the home on grounds of serious risk to the life, health and well-being of residents.' It is curious that concern for the well-being of residents did not arouse any interest in the alternatives available to them in the event of the deregistration of what had been for many years their home. In part, the explanation must surely be that there appeared to be no departmental policy for dealing with such a situation. Although the Department had appointed an officer to carry out the procedures required by the new Act in respect of the Home, there is little evidence that much thought had been given to appropriate Departmental responses in the eventuality of a voluntary home failing to meet the criteria by which satisfactory standards were now to be determined. The Department had long broken the habit of regular registration visits under previous legislation, and as a result, there was no pre-existing policy on which to fall back when dealing with the outcome of such visits. In contrast, however, the Acting Director was clear about what should be done: the Home should close. He had been in post when the Management Committee had determined at their meeting in August 1984 to close the Home. It was he who had written to the Charity Commission to negotiate the end of the Charity or the sale of the Home. He had written to the Director of Social Services to express his doubts about the future management structure of the Home. Perhaps it is not surprising that in the apparent absence of any useful policy guidelines within the Department, the Registration Officer saw the Home largely through the eyes of its Director. It is significant that in communicating her decision to the Director of Social Services on 7 December 1984 the Registration Officer said, 'In my opinion, and that of its Acting Director ... this Home falls far below acceptable standards in many important areas.' The phraseology is telling. Even if she had had an independent view it would have been difficult to withstand such conviction. The promptness with which the Acting Director's letter to the Department supporting deregistration only a day after that of the Registration Officer's was sent suggests an interpretation involving collusion of this sort. And at the very least, it was unusual for a Person-in-Charge to acquiese tamely, still less to encourage deregistration: the explanation must lie in the decisions taken by the Management Committee during August 1984.

Once the registration procedures had been put into motion, and the Home judged unfit for registration, the Directorate of the Department of Social Services was forced back into a direct relationship with the Home at last. It was a situation which the Home had been seeking to achieve at least since 1978, and the welcome given to the renewed relationship by the Acting Director in his letter of 8 December 1984 to the Director of Social Services was not entirely a response to his expectation of achieving thereby, closure:

> It is good thanks to your Department and the new legislation relating to residential establishments, that at last, firm guidelines and requirements can be stated by the ... Borough ... It is unfortunate that nine years have passed since the last official assessment.

In fact, as we have seen, the previous registration Visit had taken place six years earlier in 1978. It is important that at this stage, in the absence of any Departmental policy for the Home, the Assistant Director of the Home was able to determine the terms on which the future of the Home would be considered by the Department - namely, its sale. In the same letter, he took the opportunity to raise the possibility of the Charity purchasing a suitable property of which the Borough was about to dispose, and in particular, a nursery belonging to the Borough but located outside its boundaries. The Director of Social Services responded quickly, and on 13 December wrote to the Home, agreeing to inform the Borough of the Charity's interest in the nursery. The copy of the letter sent to the Registering Officer included a note promising to discuss the subject in the New Year.

Thus, initially, the Department was responding to a programme determined elsewhere, rather than using its influence to further a policy of its own. Discussion focussed on closure, sale and the purchase of the nursery, about which doubt soon began to emerge. Thus on 22 January 1985, the Registering Officer informed the Assistant Director that closure of the Home was imminent, but that the discussion concerning the nursery had run into the difficulty that its sale would be delayed by the Borough's insistence on putting it out to tender. On 24 January 1985, a meeting involving the Acting Director, and the Borough's Social Services and Environmental Health officers was held at which it was agreed that the Home could not go on as it was. A handwritten account of the meeting noted that the Acting Director regarded the position of the Home as 'desperate', and his preference for 'immediate removal'. The Environmental Health officers considered that a Prohibition Order should be issued as soon as possible. The Registering Officer expressed part of the dilemma: registration could be delayed in the hope of improvement, but full compliance with the fire regulations would diminish the standard of care; therefore, the Home should be closed, but there were tremendous risks attached to separating the residents.

Searching for a policy

No firm idea as to what should be done with the residents in the event of closure emerged from the meeting. The Acting Director of the Home continued in his preference for purchasing the Nursery, but the Director of Social Services pointed to the need for the sale to wait on bids because of the Borough's insistence on obtaining the market price for the property. The Director himself wondered about the possibility of buying hotel places, while the Registration Officer reminded the meeting that there were not enough places in Part 111 accommodation to absorb the residents of the Home. Nevertheless, a decision was taken to de-register the Home from 8 February 1985, and the handwritten notes of the meeting ended with a reminder to alert the financing authorities of the removal, and the allowance to the Home of two weeks for alternative arrangements to be made. On the following day (25 January 1985) the Director formally acquainted the Acting Director of the Home with these decisions in a letter, and outlined his Department's policy with regard to the Home at that stage thus:

> It would be this authority's intention to cause as little distress as possible in moving, and I am sure that my officers will give whatever help they can in advising on alternative arrangements ... Were the Home to guarantee a management committee, constitution, adequate managerial help and staffing as absolute minimal conditions for keeping the residents together, then I am sure the purchase of ... (the nursery) ... could prove the best outcome.

Thus the sale of the building in which the Home was housed was regarded as inevitable, but there was no clear and definite alternative accommodation for the residents, and only a hope that they would be kept together.

It was at this stage that a policy view began to emerge

within the Department. At first this amounted to no more than the principle of keeping the residents together. At the end of January 1985, three members of the Social Services Department visited the Home and produced a 'Progress Report'. If refurbishment of the present Home was not possible, it was argued, any alternative accommodation must ensure that residents remained together: they had come to rely on one another and saw themselves as a large family; they were more successful in supporting each other than anything which the council could provide. The Report warned that if this cohesion were to be damaged by dispersal, there would be a rapid deterioration in the condition of the more frail disabled residents. Furthermore, news of the closure had already created fear among the resident, and reassurance as soon as possible that they could remain together was a necessity.

By 12 February 1985, when a meeting was held between the newly elected Chairman of the Management Committee and the Social Services Department, it was clear that the Nursery could no longer be regarded as a suitable alternative for the Home, and it was doubtful if the local authority would agree to licence it for a change of purpose. Although the policy of keeping the residents together had been agreed, there was no clear idea within the Department as to how this could be achieved. According to the GLC Architects Department, the buildings of the present Home were basically sound, but required a great deal of work. The Registration Officer remained adamant that the Home could not be registered while the dormitories continued to exist. The Director assumed that it could not function; on the other hand, to do the basic improvements appeared to be a viable option; the choice appeared to lie between refurbishment of the present buildings, the purchase of a new building, or the development and extension of the activities with which the Charity was concerned. In elaboration of the third option, it was suggested that the Charity should cater for men and women, ethnic minorities, and adults of all ages. However, it was pointed out that this solution was precluded by the Charity's objectives. In the event, the Department offered to hold off the prohibition order, but it was made plain that the Borough would give little material help, though as a nationwide resource, the Charity might expect to attract other funds. At this stage, then, the Borough's policy appeared to be merely to reduce pressure on the Home, and encourage the Management Committee to seek elsewhere for funds for the refurbishment of the existing buildings.

However, other pressures continued to mount as the cost of refurbishment became clear. On 12 February, an electrical firm's survey revealed that the old building needed rewiring and that the plugs were overfused. It may have been this, and the Borough's lack of practical help which engendered a seige mentality at the Home. A secretarial note for 13 February 1985, reported the news that the Borough Surveyor and Architect had been refused entry at the Home by the person in charge - an indication of the beginning of the change in attitude towards the Borough on the part of the Home. On 11 March 1985, the GLC Fire Brigade Report was written. A week later, (18 March), it appeared that the Home was to pursue a policy of refurbishment. A letter from the Chairman of the Management Committee to the Director of Social Services reported that environmental health officers had served an improvement notice, and 56 days had been given by the GLC Architects and Fire Prevention Department in which the changes they required had to be effected; the Management Committee would undertake the necessary work; staffing levels at the Home had now been raised to an acceptable level; and, as a result of a death, there were now only 15 residents at the Home.

Within a month, the Management's Committee's policy, if it had ever been anything else in reality, had reverted to the original one of sale. At a Special Meeting of Trustees held on 15 April 1985, it was concluded that the costings for repair provided by an architect could not be met from funds held by the Trustees and the decision was taken to 'instruct an estate agent to look for an alternative property, within a given radius, to rehouse the residents' - the old property, according to the terms of the Trust, had to be sold by tender.

The question of finance

It is appropriate at this point to consider how the Management Committee perceived their financial situation throughout this period, for it was this which appears to have been the major determinant of their decision to sell the Home. We have already seen that the Borough's loan of £12,500, granted in 1976, had been repaid in 1983. However, after three years during which no change had been made to the level of the weekly maintenance rate, in 1984 the Home requested an increased which almost doubled the sum involved - from £50.61 at 1 April 1983 to £96.29 at 1 April 1984. The following year, the Home's accountants wrote to ask that the maintenance rate be raised again, this time to £170.00 per week. To justify this rise, it was claimed that the Home was running at a substantial weekly deficit, that it was faced with paying for £20,000 worth of repairs, and an increase in staffing levels, requirements of the Registered Homes Act 1984, and the associated code of practice. The request appears to have been granted with little question by the Borough, other than a request for the staff numbers budget for 1985-6 which was supplied on 20 May 1985. No accounts had been received by the Borough since 31 March 1983.

At a meeting on 11 June 1985 between the residents, the Home's staff, the Management Committee, and the Registration Officer to discuss the sale of the Home, and the move to a new establishment, the financial predicament of the Charity was blamed for the move. When staff raised the possibility of asking the local authority to give more time to raise money to refurbish the present Home, the Management Committee reply was that the government would not give to a small charity, that homes all over the country were having to close, and that the Charity was £50,000 'in the red'. Inevitably, the financial position of the Charity was a central feature of the Chairman's Report for 1984-5, delivered at a meeting held on 21 June 1985. This time, the deficit was said to be £39,041, and while both revenue and income were falling, the cost of maintenance had increased: to ease the situation, the maintenance rate was to be raised. Nevertheless, an attempt at fundraising had been made. But on 13 June 1985, the Chairman of the Management Committee informed the Director of Social Services that the Charity had been able to raise only £1700 by this method. By 5 September 1985, when the Assistant Director Care Services wrote to a Councillor, according to the Borough's assessment, it would have required £150,000 to make good the existing Home, which itself was valued at £450,000. However, two points need to be made in relation to the Charity's financial situation. The first is that according to papers circulated at the meeting of the Inquiry Panel on 30 October 1985, the Borough's finance officers were concerned about the apparently large number of investments and current assets which were shown in the accounts to 31 March 1983 - the last set of accounts then available to the Borough. It appeared that these assets had been accumulated as a result of a surplus of income over expenditure. The second point to notice is that when the Borough was asked to agree to a huge rise in the maintenance rate for the second year running in April 1985, to finance refurbishment as well as pay for increased staffing levels, the Management Committee had already decided to sell the Home and seek another property.

Opposition to sale

Although the Borough had firmly adopted the policy of pressing for the residents to be kept together in the event of the Home's sale, and attempted to shield the Charity by delaying the application of the health and safety regulations in the hope that a policy of refurbishment would be pursued, once the decision to sell had become known, pressures from other sources arose which affected not only the Charity but also the Borough. However these pressures affected the two organisations in different ways. Whereas the Charity became increasingly intransigent in its attachment to the policy of sale and purchase, the Borough was forced to adopt a more directly interventionist approach, especially when dispersal of the residents appeared to be a danger, and to extend its policy to include the requirement that the Home should remain within the Borough's boundaries. As a result, Borough and Home came into conflict, and those employees of the Social Services Department who had made informal links with the Home and were now elected members of its Management Committee became identified with that Committee's policy of sale, and as a consequence, found themselves in conflict with their employers.

The first source of pressure on the Charity was the attitude of its employees at the Home. On 11 June 1985, a meeting between residents, staff, the officers of the Social Services Department who were also members of the Management Committee and were present in that capacity, and the Registration Officer for the Home, was held to discuss the situation. It is a mark of the divorce between Management Committee and Borough that the fact that the meeting took place remained unknown to the Social Services Directorate until unofficial minutes were sent anonymously to a Councillor two months later: on 15 August 1985, a copy of the minutes was passed by that Councillor to the Director. Most striking of all was the failure of the Registration Officer to report the meeting to the Department, even though she was declared, in a letter from the Assistant Director Care Services on 5 September 1985, to the Councillor who had received the minutes, to have been there as a representative of the Department, not in her capacity as the wife of the Chairman of the Management Committee. It appears to be the case that her identity with the policy of sale, already in evidence before Christmas 1984, and manifest throughout the discussions on the Home's future held in January and February 1985, had been strengthened by her husband's position in the Charity and his continued support for the policy of sale. Once a breach began to emerge between the Charity and the Department, her loyalty, like that of Departmental employees on the Management Committee lay with the Charity. Because of the informality and anonymity of the minutes, as well as the way in which they were used to strengthen opposition to the Charity's policy of sale, their content has to be treated with caution. It seems safe to conclude, however, that the residents and staff were united in their opposition to the proposed move.

The puzzle as to why the sale was necessary, when already the Home had been refurbished to the point at which it satisfied the health, safety and fire regulations, and all that was left to be done was to provide single rooms and decent wash basins, was a question raised by staff, and only confusingly answered by Committee members. The Committee's case appears to have rested partly on the threat that the Director of Social Services could still close the Home at any time, and drag off the residents to homes for the elderly - an unlikely possibility given the declared lack of space in Part 111 accommodation. Their case also appeared to rest in part on the requirement that 'this business has to be viable'. In this connection the debt of £50,000 was stressed, and the possibility of raising funds without a sale dismissed: the Director of Social Services had given no hope of an improvement grant; the government would not give money to a small charity, as any establishment with fewer than 200 residents was not viable and homes all over the country were having to close. In the circumstances, it was pointless to consult the residents since they had no choice in the matter. A minibus would be purchased so that residents could be brought back for visits to maintain their links with the Borough. The decision to move was a perfectly proper one, arrived at in consultation with the Charity Commission. Members of the Committee appear to have taken the view that in fact, the residents were lucky that the Home had not closed before Christmas when dispersal would have been likely; that this had not happened was due to their own efforts - although they were employees of the Department which had served the closure notice, they had worked hard for an extension.

The unresolved dichotomy noted in the anonymous minutes between the improvements made to the Home and the insistence on selling it, reappeared in the Chairman's Report for 1984-5 on the Charity. This serenely noted that the Home now met health and safety requirements; that although two residents had died in the course of the year, a new one was expected to arrive and it was hoped that other new arrivals were a possibility; that a satisfactory appointment was about to be made to the post of care manager on a permanent basis; and that the life of the Home had continued to run satisfactorily, with day outings, regular attendance at the Day Centre and Church, and the holding of a rummage sale attended by the Mayor. Yet they had searched for an alternative Home and had now been successful.

In the circumstances it is not surprising that representatives of voluntary and community groups began to join staff in questioning the activities of the Management Committee and also the relatively low profile adopted by the Local Authority. In fairness to both, it must be admitted that the closure of a home for the deaf and the removal of the residents to another home, and even their dispersal among a number of different establishments, was not unknown: in the late 1970s, RNID had adopted both approaches in its effort to slim down its involvement with residential care provision. Indeed, in 1978, RNID had adopted that very policy against which the Borough's Social Services Department had set itself from the outset - the dispersal of residents to homes for the elderly.

By July, there is increasing evidence of wariness on the part of the Management Committee in its relationship with the Borough. On 9 July, the Assistant Director Care Services was informed that the Management Committee was reluctant to allow an independent interpreter to interview residents, and that they had actually refused a request for such a visit. The Management Committee began to develop a seige mentality as individuals and organisations outside the Charity and the Social Services Department were drawn into the conflict. On 13 July 1985, the Chairman of the Management Committee informed the Director of Social Services that negotiations were underway for the purchase for a hotel well beyond the Borough's boundary, that the local M.P. had become involved in, and associated himself with the opposition of the Home's staff to the move; yet the move had been made inevitable by the failure of the Charity's fund-raising efforts to bring in more than £1700. On the same day, after hearing a rumour that the Management Committee intended to sell up and disperse the women, the Director of Social Services, who said that he had previously assumed that they would upgrade the present buildings, asked the Assistant Director Care Services to investigate the Home. A report was required for the meeting of the Integrated Planning Group for Disability on 20 September, and that group wished an officer and a representative of the local Association for disabled people to be involved in the inquiry.

As opposition to the sale grew, the Management Committee came under increasing pressure, and its members' behaviour became more and more questionable. Symptomatic of this development was the Chairman's letter to the local M.P. on 16 July 1985, in which he justified the sale as a solution to the problems of the Home by downgrading the importance of the locality of the Home to the residents, arguing that only three came from the Borough in any case, and that because of their age, their deafness, and the way in which the Home had been administered until recently, there had been little integration of the residents into the local community. While this was superficially true, he must have known that all the residents had lived in the locality for many years; and if he had known anything about the deaf community he would have been aware of the importance of familiarity as an aid to communication, and of the fact that though like most deaf people they had failed to integrate into hearing community, they had established valuable links with the deaf community. Furthermore, the opposition of the residents to the move was to be discounted, he argued, because it had been stimulated by staff who had also orchestrated local opposition because they had 'a vested interest in preserving their jobs locally'. It was a viewpoint which ignored the fact that few in old age face the prospect of upheaval with equanimity, and that the prospect of job loss is bound to cause considerable anxiety at a time of high unemployment, especially in an area such as the Borough, which suffered disproportionately from unemployment. Moreover, some dissembling was required to propose closure as the only serious alternative to sale, since it had been made clear in November 1984 that the Charity Commissioners would not countenance closure. However, the charge that 'The interest now shown by you and the local community has come too late' was timely. As we have seen, the difficulties of the Home had been festering for almost a decade, and despite a particularly urgent cry for help in 1978, no material help had been forthcoming either then, or even when the Borough itself officially recognised the Home's plight.

Throughout August and September 1985, pressures on both the Charity and the Department of Social Services continued to mount. On 15 August, the Director was sent a letter by a Councillor suggesting that he and his Department were not receiving unbiased advice from officers, and with the letter was enclosed the anonymous minutes of the meeting of 11 June. The next day a representative of a local organisation for the elderly stressed the interests of the residents: in view of the number of years they had lived in the Borough, their considerable social contacts in the locality, the fact that they had signed a letter to the Management Committee expressing opposition to the move even though they had visited and admired the hotel which was their intended home, selling the Home appeared to be the wrong policy, though it had to be admitted that the Management Committee had inherited a difficult problem. On 19 August, a local community action news sheet included a report on the Home and the action taken by the voluntary association for the elderly.

The effect of the developing pressure on the Department of Social Services was to increase the activity surrounding the establishment of an investigative panel and to put pressure on the Management Committee to change its policy of sale. On 3 September 1985, the Director expressed to the Chairman of the Management Committee, the Social Services Committee's considerable concern at the sale, informed him of the existence of the review panel, reminded him of his promise to keep the residents together in the Borough, and expressed doubts about the compliance of residents with the scheme. In fact, there is no record of any unequivocal undertaking by the Charity to keep the residents together in the Borough. It seems likely that the Director gained the impressioon that this was their policy as a result of the Management Committee's refurbishing activities. It was now Borough policy to seek to delay the sale until the Panel's investigation was completed. At the same time, however, the Social Services Directorate was concerned to defend itself against the charge that its personnel were out of control. Thus, on 5 September 1985, the Assistant Director Care Services wrote to a Councillor to explain that those officers who had been elected to the Home's Management Committee had not asked permission to be associated with the Home in this way because it was the accepted custom for staff to engage in such activities in their spare time.

If the external pressures which developed during the summer of 1985 stimulated an increasingly interventionist response by the Department of Social Services, it was also responsible for increasing intransigence on the part of the Management Committee, who now began to ignore both the best interests of the residents and local opinion. That this was so emerged clearly in relation to the issue of the residents' wishes regarding the move to another home and another district. On 30 August 1985, the Registration Officer informed the Director that an Independent Interpreter adopted by the Trustees had interviewed the residents with all the staff present, and they had agreed that they wished to stay together, while some of the staff would go to the new home as well. However, it soon emerged that this note signalled the beginning of a certain amount of evasive behaviour on the part of the Management Committee to ease the sale and purchase procedure. On 5 September, the Independent Interpreter's misgivings about her role in the meeting held on 30 August were such that she felt obliged to describe the process of consultation which had taken place to the Social Services Directorate. She had been required to relay a letter from the Management Committee and, under their instructions, 'ask the residents whether they wanted to move to new accommodation ... or to residential care in their own particular local authority'. She had to communicate what each party had said as accurately and objectively as possible. Most of the residents wished to remain where they were, in an area which they knew well and regarded as home. However, the Management Committee repeatedly stressed that this was not a choice open to them. The Independent Interpreter concluded that the residents should be consulted in less intimidating conditions. So incensed were the Management Committee by her disclosure of the meeting that when the Independent Interpreter sought to claim her fees, the Committee's Secretary wrote to charge her with 'breach of confidentiality' for disclosing information to 'outside bodies': doubt was cast on whether the work had been carried out satisfactorily, and the question of fees would have to go to Committee for consideration. (It must be remembered that the Management Committee's Secretary was an officer of the Social Services Department.) In the face of this unpleasant rebuff, the Independent Interpreter sought the help of the Assistant Director Care Services on 6 October 1985, in drafting a reply, to be checked by the Borough's legal department, in which she argued, among other things, that in this matter the Borough could not be regarded as an 'outside body'. On 18 October, the Registration Officer was asked to account for the discrepancy between her own report of the meeting of 30 August, and that sent to the Director by the Independent Interpreter. There is no record of an explanation.

Sale, purchase and move

Evasiveness was also evident in the Committee's handling of the suitability of the Hotel premises in which the residents were to be accommodated on the sale of the Home. Justifying the sale of the Home on the grounds that it would prevent the closure of the Charity, which had once seemed inevitable and imminent, the Chairman of the Management Committee, in a letter to the Director on 13 September 1985, contrasted the dramatically below standard nature of the accommodation available in the present Home as assessed under the new registration Act, despite the work undertaken to bring it up to the standard required under the health and safety legislation, with the Hotel to which residents were to move which already complied with many of the regulations. [5] To bring the Home up to registration standard was beyond the means of the Charity. In contrast, the Hotel afforded privacy, a delightful environment, and a high standard of decoration and furnishings. Resources were available in the area for the deaf, though the maintenance of links with the Borough would be ensured by the purchase of a minibus which could ferry residents to the Day Centre and Church. If the quality of the lives of the residents was to improve, there was no alternative to the policy of sale and removal.

However, a fortnight later, (28 September 1985), a telephone message from the Representative of local people with disabilities, who was on the Borough's Social Services Committee, reported that the Hotel was not up to registration standard. Further telephone messages that day and the following day reported that the Registration Officer for the new Local Authority had no knowledge of an application for registration: the Hotel was known and would require 'substantial adaptation'. On 31 September the Area Organiser of the district in which the Hotel was situated telephoned to say that the District Fire Officer had not heard of the move, there had been no attempt to comply with the regulations, no plans had been seen, and conversion would be necessary. As evidence accumulated of the disturbing nature of the situation which was developing, the Assistant Director Care Services wrote to the Chairman of the Management Committee on 1 November 1985, to ask for reassurance in view of the fact that the Hotel was not yet registered, though completion was to take place on 11 November. Meanwhile, on 5 November, a handwritten note reported that the Home's Registration Officer (and wife of the Chairman of the Management Committee) 'in her capacity as a member of the Management Committee', had met a representative of the new Local Authority to discuss the move: as no application for registration had been made, it had not been possible to contact all the relevant bodies from whom assessments would be required. It was not until 7 January 1986, when the residents had been settled in the Hotel for two months, that the Chairman of the Management Committee chose to reply to the Assistant Director regarding registration, in a letter which did not mention registration as such but concentrated on contrasting favourably the Hotel with the Home in terms of safety and comfort. The interests of residents were said to be well protected, their welfare assured, and the standards of safety and accommodation at the Hotel were in all respects superior to those at the Home, save for the absence of a lift between floors, and the installation of a lift was in hand. The risks to which residents were exposed were no greater in the Hotel than at the Home, and the residents were all 'evidently happy'. In the absence of any further information from the Management Committee, the Assistant Director Care Services wrote to the new Local Authority's Director of Social Services on 26 April 1986 to ask if the Hotel now satisfied the conditions of registration and if it were now registered. The reply he received on 4 June 1986, vindicated the agitation which had been aroused by the removal of the residents, justified the Borough's fear concerning the competence of the Management Committee, and raised questions about the motives of the Committee members, especially those employed by the Borough's Department of Social Services. The Hotel did not satisfy the conditions for registration, and as considerable work was still outstanding in respect of fire precaution requirements, it was difficult to forecast when registration was likely to take place. If the Trustees had made contact with the new Local Authority regarding the purchase of the Hotel, they would have been made aware that the property did not come anywhere near meeting the requirements of the Registered Homes Act 1984, or of the Authority's own Departmental Operational Guidelines. Thus the assurances given to the Borough on 7 January either were given in ignorance, or were intended to mislead. Whichever was the case, it appeared that the residents were not in good hands.

Evasion and thoughtlessness regarding the immediate interests of residents also appear to have characterised the Management Committee's handling of the move from Home to Hotel. The issue of the date on which the move was to take place was of moment not only to the registering authority in its pursuit of a policy of delay, but also to the Borough and other local authorities as sponsors of residents at the Home, and as such with responsibility for determining the wishes of residents regarding the move from Home to Hotel. Furthermore, there were the relatives of residents who were to be faced with maintaining a relationship with, and checking on the welfare of loved ones living in a new location. Whatever else may be said about the Home, relationships between relatives and residents seem to have been maintained there to a quite unusual degree compared with other homes for the deaf. Responsibility for keeping other local authorities informed of the Charity's intention was undertaken by the Borough as the registering authority, while negotiating with residents was the clear duty of the Management Committee. In the event, the increasing reluctance of the Management Committee to divulge fully its plans to the Social Services Department made it difficult for the Borough to discharge its responsibility to other local authorities, and there is no evidence to suggest that the Management Committee consulted the relatives of residents or kept them informed as to the date of the move.

As early as 25 January 1985, it is clear from a handwritten account that the Social Services Directorate was aware of the importance of informing financing authorities about the likelihood of deregistration, and on the same day, the Director reported to the Acting Director of the Home that he was informing the various financing authorities for individual residents immediately. It soon became clear that other local authorities were as ambivalent as the Borough as to where the best interests of the residents lay - in good quality care provided directly themselves, or in the little community within which residents had lived for so long. Thus on 5 February 1985, a local authority wrote to explain that while its residents could be housed within their native boundaries, they were free to remain within their little community if a good standard of care could be guaranteed. It was not until 13 September 1985, well after the decision had been taken by the Management Committee to respond to the threat of closure associated with deregistration by selling the Home and moving to the Hotel, that its Chairman wrote to the Borough's Director of Social Services to report that the move would take place in November 1985, and that each local authority should be asked to consult their residents and to make alternative arrangements for those who did not want to go to the Hotel. On 24 September, a list of residents and their sponsoring authorities was drawn up by the Social Services Department with whom consultations had to be held. Three days later (27 September 1985), the Assistant Director Care Services wrote to tell directors with residents at the Home that his Department was to hold talks with all residents, and to ask for such action to be approved. On 9 October, the Assistant Director informed the Director of Social Services that most local authorities had agreed that the Borough should hold consultations with their residents, though two wished to send their own interpreter. A collaborative approach was adopted by the Borough towards local authorities intending to utilise the services of their own interpreters in the consultation exercise. Thus, on 15 October 1985, a handwritten unsigned note reported on arrangements to be made with another London Borough for discussions concerning interviews with residents.

There was still no firm information regarding the sale of the Home and the date of removal to the Hotel. As late as 18 October 1985, the Assistant Director Care Services had to write to the Chairman of the Management Committee asking for confirmation of the sale and the date on which the move was to take place. It seems clear that the relatives of residents were excluded from discussions on and information about the move. On the same day, the Director reported to the Assistant Director that the daughter of one of the residents, who had been appointed Receiver by the Court of Protection of which her mother was a ward, was never notified in either capacity - as daughter or Receiver - of the move, and said that residents did not want to move: the Home had been sold and residents and staff were to move on 8 November 1985. As late as 24 October, the Management Committee's Secretary informed her employer, the Director of Social Services, that the Borough's three residents would be moved on 11 November 1985. The following day, the Assistant Director wrote to the Chairman of the Management Committee reporting the agreement of other local authorities that Borough representatives should interview residents to ascertain their wishes. On 29 October, the Director informed the Assistant Director by telephone that he had had a letter from the Home informing him that the move was to take place on 11 November. However, on the same day, a telephone call was received from the daughter of a resident informing the Assistant Director that she had heard from an agency nurse at the Home, that the move was to take place on 8 November. This was the second time within a fortnight that the Social Services Department had heard from a relative of a date for removal which was earlier than the official one. News of the earlier removal date soon reached other local authorities with residents at the Home, and on 29 October a telephone message from the London borough which wished to interview its own residents suggested the urgency of planning joint interviews of residents with the Borough.

The Management Committee continued to stress the importance of the completion date of 11 November, but became ambiguous with regard to the date of removal. Thus on 30 October, the Chairman of the Management Committee informed the Assistant Director of no more than the reality of the move and the completion date. Yet on 5 November, a hand written note indicates that the wife of the Chairman of the Management Committee (and the Borough's Registration Officer for the Home) had met a representative of the new Local Authority 'to discuss the move which is to take place tomorrow'. In the event, the arrangements for residents to be interviewed before the move, and made jointly between the Management Committee, the Borough's newly appointed deaf specialist Senior Social Worker, and his counterpart from the other London borough which wished to maintain direct responsibility for ascertaining the views of its residents, were aborted by the Management Committee: the two interpreters arrived to see the residents assembled in the coach and departing for the Hotel.

By no means all relatives of residents had been able to find out even unofficially about the move, still less its date. On 29 November, a letter was received by the Social Services Department from a woman who explained that she was accustomed to visit her half sister at the Home every other week, that she had discovered that the residents had moved, and that she had been unable to find out her half sister's new address. At least one director of social services whose department sponsored a resident at the Home, was perplexed at the lack of news regarding the wishes of residents - a perplexity which increased as news began to seep out that the Hotel in its present condition was not registerable. On 23 November, the Director received a letter from a colleague in the Home Counties who complained that he had received no account of the interviews with residents which had been promised and that anxiety had been aroused by the information from the new Local Authority that the Hotel did not meet fire regulation standards: if their resident was unhappy they would make other arrangements for her, but if she had settled in happily, she could stay where she was as she had been at the Home for 25 years. Thus the secrecy surrounding the precise date of removal prevented financing authorities from conducting interviews directly or by proxy with their residents to ascertain their views on the move, and caused uncertainty and worry to relatives, especially those who visited the Home regularly.

Media and councillors

The extraordinary game of subterfuge in which the members of the Management Committee indulged is difficult to explain within the confines of the evidence available in the Social Services Department's records. However, two related factors may help to explain their behaviour. The first was the evidence of increasing media interest in the affair, and the second was the growing determination on the part of the Social Services Department, partly as a result of pressure from Council members, to act to delay the move. The two factors were inter-related in the sense that television and press reports stimulated activity by Council members, while in turn, their activity aroused the interest of news reporters. Media interest in the issue had begun on 19 August 1985, at a local level with a report in the local community action newspaper on the Home and the intervention of the local Voluntary Association for the Elderly. By 10 October, the Borough was sufficiently alarmed at both the behaviour of the Management Committee and the groundswell of local and elected opinion, to issue a news release: the sale of the Home was unfair, and local councillors were mounting a lastditch attempt to prevent it; the Leader of the Council had written to the Trustees to assert that the interests of the residents were not being taken into account; and the Director of Social Services was not satisfied that residents had not been intimidated.

At one stage, media interest prevented interviews with some residents to determine their views about the move. On 15 October 1985, an unsigned handwritten note recorded a telephone call from a neighbouring London borough reporting unhappiness regarding the possibility of their deaf specialist social worker interviewing their three residents on the following day while a television crew was present. A telex report dated 16 October 1985 by the Broadcasting Reporting Service indicates that the event in question had been televised for Local News. The gist of the item had been that the Charity was insisting that the 'Disabled Women' had to leave London for another area and that the 15 residents had written to the Chairman of the Management Committee saying that they did not want to move. The programme included interviews with a resident and an interpreter, the Leader of the Council, and the local M.P. Although the Chairman of the Management Committee was not interviewed, he was reported as insisting that the residents were going to a better life, and that the move had been made inevitable by the Borough's requirement that the Charity undertake £100,000 worth of improvements. The Borough's insistence that it had offered help with the improvements was reported, as was that of the Secretary of the Management Committee that the move would go ahead. Such public altercation must have ruined relationships already soured, between the Borough and the Management Committee.

Councillors tended to respond to pressures from local community groups and in turn sought responses from Council officers. On 18 September 1985, the local Voluntary Association for the Elderly sent to one Councillor, who passed it on to another as well as to officers of the Social Services Department, copies of letters sent to the Charity Commission pleading that it should make representations to prevent or delay the sale of the Home. On 30 September 1985, the Leader of the Council wrote to the Assistant Director Care Services to report that the Borough's representative for people with disabilities had suggested that he, the Leader of the Council, should write to the Charity Commission: he was willing to do so, or make other representations which might delay a decision and give the Panel time to conduct their Inquiry. Another Councillor wrote to the Director on 10 October 1985, to note that the Charity Commissioners did not appear to be responding, and asking what else the Council could do to be helpful.

The Charity Commission

With the failure of direct pressure on the Management Committee, and of informal links to further its policy, the Council sought to bring pressure to bear indirectly on the Management Committee, by seeking to persuade other organisations which might have an influence, of the justice of its policies. It appeared at the outset that the obvious focus for pressure to influence the Management Committee to moderate their policy of sale to at least one of delay, was the Charity Commission. In 1984, the Charity Commission had prevented the closure of the Charity, but it is clear from correspondence between the Commissioners and the Acting Director of the Home that in general the relationship between the two had been neither close nor demanding. When replying, on 28 August 1984, to the request that the Charity should be allowed to close, Commissioners urged discussion, and reminded the Acting Director that no accounts had been received from the Charity since 1969-70. On 30 October 1984, the Acting Director replied by enclosing the accounts for the previous three years, reporting the need for a new Committee, and promising to visit the Commission to discuss the Home's problems. In the circumstances, perhaps it is surprising that the Commissioners did not request all the accounts since 1970: a thorough investigation of the recent financial history of the Home would appear to have been essential for an adequate assessment of its current plight. In the following month it became clear that the overriding interest of the Commission was in the Home's viability as a charity. On 14 November, the Commission wrote to the Acting Director stressing that the Home could not close if there were beneficiaries, and suggesting that if the present Trustees could not manage the Charity, others should be found, and suitable people coopted from the Local Authority. As the existing constitution of the Charity was now out of date the Commission promised to draft a new scheme. The Commission thus refused to allow the Management Committee to escape from its misery by closure, and insisted on an alternative solution. Its own contribution to the process was to be constitutional modernisation. That Charity Commissioners were not concerned with standards of care or the welfare of beneficiaries emerged clearly from the correspondence between them and those who sought to delay or prevent the sale of the Home. Thus on 18 September 1985, in their reply to the Borough's Representative of people with disabilities, a Commissioner pointed out that as the Charity was a national one the Management Committee could move it wherever they liked, and were bound to act in the interest of future as well as present beneficiaries - the interest of beneficiaries was clearly assumed to be identified with the existence of the Charity, not the type of care provided by it. The Commissioner further explained that as the decision to sell appeared to have been taken in good faith, and in making it no breach of trust seemed to have occurred, the Commission could not set the decision aside. It was a reply which had already been sent on 13 September 1985 to the Director of Social Services: as the Charity was national it could be located anywhere, and the Trustees were required to obtain the best price for the sale of the Home. In his letter of 17 September 1985, to the Commission the Chairman of the local Voluntary Association for the Elderly argued the importance of customary surroundings for those in old age and with communication problems, the absence of any time limit under the Registered Homes Act for the implementation of regulations concerning standards, and the elimination of the Charity's financial problems by the raising of the maintenance rate. He pointed out that the unwillingness of the Management Committee to provide information merely created doubt, and that its members were behaving in this unhelpful and worrying way because they knew they had the support of the Commission. But the Commission remained unmoved.

Council members also sought to influence the Charity Commission in the hope that the sale would be delayed at the very least. The Leader of the Council wrote to the Assistant Director Care Services on 30 September 1985, offering to write to the Charity Commission if it was thought that this would be helpful, and do anything else which would delay the move. The next day he duly wrote to the Commission attempting to interpret their regulations of 16 July 1984 (Section 8) - namely that 'Trustees must exercise reasonable care in all matters relating to the charity and must always keep in mind the interests of the charity ... (and) must act with complete fairness between beneficiaries ...' in such a way that the Charity and its interests were synonymous with the interests of current beneficiaries. Neither this argument nor a plea regarding the helplessness of the residents in making their views known to a hearing world, and the desirability of delaying the sale until an investigation of its consequences for the residents had been completed, could sway the Commissioners. Despite the rebuffs, the Council persisted in seeking to exert pressure in this way. On 18 October, the Assistant Director Care Services suggested to another Council member who had been enquiring as to what might be done, that he should add his voice to those asking the Charity Commission to delay the sale.

However, by the latter part of October, it was clear that no support could be expected from this quarter, and as a last resort, help was sought from organisations for people with disabilities which might be expected to have influence with the Charity's Management Committee in an attempt to effect the policy of delay. Thus the Director of Social Services wrote to a national voluntary organisation for the deaf, and a national association for people with disabilities asking them to urge the Management Committee to delay until the Council's own inquiry was complete. Whatever the impact of these communications upon their recipients, they had no discernible effect on the actions of the Management Committee.

The Panel of Inquiry

Despite the agitation in which the Borough engaged to prevent the sale of the Home, there was never any willingness to offer the Charity the practical aid which would have obviated the claim of financial necessity as the reason for the move. As we have seen, from the outset, in his discussions during January and February 1985, with the Chairman of the Management Committee, the Director of Social Services failed to respond with the possibility of Borough help, beyond delaying the application of the closure notice. And this position was maintained through the summer months of that year as the likelihood of sale and removal became increasingly obvious. For example, the records for 4 September 1985, contain evidence that the Social Services Department was investigating the limit of its mandatory obligations with regard to the Home's residents: the duty to provide residential accommodation under Section 21, and to promote the welfare of the Deaf and Dumb under Section 29 of the National Assistance Act 1948 were noted as the statutory responsibilities laid upon the Council.

No doubt the investigation by the Panel of Inquiry was prompted by the growing agitation by local pressure groups and Councillors that the Social Services Department should 'do something' about the Charity: in such circumstances, to determine the bottom line was essential. But it soon became clear that little more than the absolute minimum of help required under statute was to be expected. On 5 September 1985, replying to the request of the Council's Leader for an explanation of the behaviour of the Council officers on the Home's Management Committee, the Assistant Director Care Services pointed out that the Department was required to do no more for the residents than provide alternative accommodation in homes for the elderly or disabled. Yet pressure from outside the Department for stronger measures to ensure the delay or prevention of the Home's removal increased rapidly as the completion date grew nearer. On 7 October 1985, the Leader of the Council wrote to the Director and the Borough Solicitor seeking advice on further action, including legal action. Two weeks later, on 28 October, the Borough's representative for people with disabilities telephoned with the news that the hotel was not up to registration standard, and urged that in the circumstances the Borough should refuse to allow the Home to move. Three days later (31 October 1985) the Area Organiser responsible for registering the Hotel with the new Local Authority telephoned to report that conversion would be necessary and that no attempt to comply with the regulations had been made: should the new Local Authority stop the move or would such action cause the Borough problems? No response seems to have been made to this suggestion by the Borough, though within a week (5 November 1985) it was noted that if the new Local Authority were to allow the move 'they would be putting vulnerable people at risk' and there is evidence in this handwritten note to indicate that the

Department was in the process of seeking an injunction to prevent the move. The injunction was never issued because the Department was not prepared to undertake the Charity's responsibilities and was advised that such a move would not succeed. The Borough's ambivalence was admitted by the Director in a letter of 11 October 1985 to the Chairman of the local Voluntary Association for the Elderly; while insisting that he had often made it plain that the Council wished to retain the facility within the Borough and would help the Trustees to keep it there, he agreed that no doubt the Trustees felt that the Council was not in a position to say how much financial assistance it would render. In the circumstances, the Borough's insistence, in response to the Management Committee's revelation on a television news item on 16 October 1985 that £100,000 worth of improvements were required by the Home, that the Council had offered help, could at best be called dissembling. The only help offered had been a stay of execution.

The limitations of the new Registration Act became apparent in the course of the dispute over the future of the Home in 1985. Gradually, it became clear that faced with a recalcitrant charity, the local authority's only option was to force closure, once a policy of delay and persuasion were no longer applicable, and, if it wished to retain the facility within its own boundaries, to assume total responsibility for the residents. As it became clear that only an injunction would prevent the removal of the Home, a final attempt to delay the move was made by initiating an investigation into the whole affair. That investigation itself demonstrated the restricted nature of the powers of the local authority over a charity. As early as 13 July 1985, when it became clear that the Management Committee did not intend to continue with the policy of upgrading the Home which had already brought it up to Health and Safety standards, the Director of Social Services told his Assistant Director Care Services to investigate the Home and to involve in the Inquiry others, including a representative of the Borough's Association for people with disabilities. Taxed by the Leader of the Council as to the Department's response to the situation, the Assistant Director Care Services was able to point to the Inquiry, on 16 August 1985. As a result of pressure from the Leader of the Council, and the deliberations of the Social Services Committee on 2 September 1985, the Inquiry was placed in the hands of members of a Panel. And from then on, the Council's object was to persuade the Management Committee to delay the sale until the Panel had completed its investigation. At the end of September and the beginning of October (30 September and 1 October) the idea of the Panel was welcomed by Councillors. October 1985 was taken up with establishing the Panel which ultimately consisted of the Assistant Director Care Services (Chair), the Representative of the Borough's Association for people with disabilities, the Chairman of the local Association for the Elderly, the newly appointed Senior Social Worker (Deaf), the Manager of an Area Office, one of the Borough's finance officers, and an outside Assessor.

The decision to set up the Panel was taken before its legal status had been determined. On 2 October, the Assistant Director Care Services told a prospective member of the Panel that a meeting was to be held shortly with the Borough's Legal Department to determine the legality of the investigation. A week later, he had to inform the Director, that the Borough Solicitor had assured him that the Department had no statutory power to carry out a formal investigation since there was no evidence of crime or malpractice. As a consequence, the Assistant Director was unsure how to proceed. Nevertheless, letters continued to be sent to outside organisations in the hope that they would influence the Management Committee to delay the removal of the Home until the investigation had been concluded: for example, on 23 October, such a letter was written by the Director to the Director General of a national association for the deaf.

Initially, the Panel urged every measure to prevent the removal of the Home, including an injunction, until its work was complete. But the Borough proved to be unwilling to assign the resources which an injunction would have entailed. Once the move to the Hotel had taken place, the scope of the Panel's investigation as well as its role, inevitably, was reduced. At that stage, two issues arose for consideration. The first was concerned with policy for deaf people in the Borough. The immediate concern was with the interests and well being of the residents, and how these should best be eliminated. But there was the further long term question of whether the facility should be used by the Borough in the future, and if not, how acceptable alternative arrangements could be made. In response to the first problem, the initial requisite appeared to be for members of the Panel to visit the Hotel and establish how well residents had settled into their new accommodation. However, it soon became clear that even this limited undertaking was beyond the investigative powers of the Panel. Arrangements were made with the wife of the Chairman of the Management Committee (and former Registration Officer for the Home) by the Senior Social Worker (Deaf) for three Panel members - himself, the Borough's Representative for people with disabilities, and the outside Assessor - to visit the Hotel on 9 December. Five days before the visit was due to take place, the Chairman of the Management Committee denied knowledge of the arrangement and refused Panel members entry to the Hotel. Only the Senior Social Worker (Deaf) would be allowed inside, in his capacity of specialist social worker, not Panel member, to talk to the three residents for whom the Borough had financial responsibility. Although this visit took place more than a month after the move from the Home, some of the residents had still not unpacked their suitcases. Although care staff at the Hotel attributed this behaviour to laziness, the specialist Social Worker felt that from conversation with residents who were huddled together in one part of the lounge, an alternative explanation could have been that some residents were under the impression that they had come to the Hotel for a short stay.

It was striking that despite the importance attached to the absence of care staff with manual communication skills by the Registration Officer in her Report on the Home, the Management Committee had still not acquired staff who could communicate in sign language with residents a year after that Report was made. At this stage, it seemed clear that while the Health and Safety Regulations were not met by the Hotel, there had been an improvement in the quantity, but not the quality of staff, and in the comfort and privacy available to residents - furniture, carpets and curtains were abundant, and most residents were in single or double bedded rooms with private bathrooms attached. At the second visit of the Senior Social Worker (Deaf) to the Hotel the newly appointed Person in Charge welcomed his services as an interpreter, made extensive use of his communication skills, suggested his membership of the Management Committee, and promised that she and her staff would attend a three day course on manual communication. While this seemed to signal the possibility of improvement in the care regime, the Hotel still fell substantially below registration standards in other respects. At that point it seemed clear to the Panel that discussion about future policy regarding residential care for deaf people in the Borough had to await the resolution of the Hotel's difficulties. Much would depend upon the degree of influence which the Senior Social Worker (Deaf) could exert on the Management Committee, and the degree to which the new Local Authority was prepared to take an interventionist approach to its relationship with the Hotel.

The second issue on which it was decided that the Panel should concentrate was the role played in decision making regarding the Home, its management and the move to the Hotel by officers of the Social Services Department. It had become a matter for concern among both elected members of the Council and the Social Services Directorate that Council officers in their private capacity had created informal links between

Department and Home which were used not to transmit Council policies, but to buttress already established Management Committee policies, which were widely regarded in the Borough, both inside and outside the Department, as being detrimental to the interests of the residents. Of particular interest was the part played by officers in the evasion which marked the behaviour of the Management Committee towards the Department from June 1985 until the move to the Hotel took place in the following November. The tradition of informal links between Council and Voluntary Home had assumed a large measure of convergence of interest, and that where there were differences such links would be used to press the Council's point of view. The possibility that interests would diverge sharply, and that in any ensuing dispute, officers of the council would not only side with the Voluntary Agency rather than their employers, but furthermore, would effectively block the possibility of the implementation of Council policy, never seems to have been considered. The history of the relationship between the Borough and the Home shattered the cosy illusions of tradition in this respect, and marked out the dangers inherent in a system in which control over voluntary bodies indirectly dependent upon public funds was based on such informal arrangements. It seems likely that problems have rarely if ever arisen in the past, either because the interests of council and voluntary agency genuinely have not been at issue, or because councils which rely on this mechanism have not bothered to formulate a policy with regard to the homes in question, or have not sought to implement their policies.

Indeed, the very informality of the situation was such that the Panel was ineffective even with regard to this aspect of its inquiry. Once the Charity was no longer within the Borough's boundaries, the only means of obtaining the necessary information was to ask the officers who had been involved with the Charity to attend a Panel meeting to explain their behaviour. Letters were sent on 5 December 1985 to the Home's former Registration Officer (and wife of the Management Committee's Chairman) and to the officer from the Research and Development Unit, to attend a Panel meeting on 12 December. In both cases it was made clear that this would not be a substitute for any of the Council's procedures, and that trade union representation would be welcome. The response of the trade union Branch Officer on behalf of the Research and Development Unit's officer on 9 December accurately pinpointed the weakness of the Panel's position: the officer in question had had contact with the Home only as a private individual, and the Borough had no right to conduct an inquiry into a national charity. Neither of the officers concerned presented themselves at the Panel meeting.

In late April the following year (26 April 1986) another attempt was made to convene a Panel meeting to be attended by the three officers still in the Council's employ, who had been involved with the Home's Management Committee - the officer from the Research and Development Unit, the former Registration Officer of the Home, and the Officer in Charge of the Day Centre attended by the residents of the Home. The purpose of the exercise was described as being to help to develop

> clear guidelines regarding the relationship between officers of the Department and voluntary organisations who are providing a service to vulnerable client groups within the Borough or to clients who are the responsibility of this authority.

At the same time, a letter stating the same objective was sent to the Chairman of the Management Committee, and included a request for copies of the minutes and agendum of the Committee's meeting, annual reports and minutes of the Charity's AGM, and the names and designations of the Management Committee members for the period 1983-1986, as well as details of the information and notice of the move given to relatives of residents. Once more, the powerlessness of the Panel and the Department of Social Services was exposed.

On 2 May 1986, the trade union reply on behalf of the Home's former Registration Officer, referring to the possibility of a conflict of interest - an issue which had been raised by the Department - pointed out that the Department's staff code referred only to employment with other organisations in this respect. On 12 May, the union reply on behalf of the Person in Charge of the Day Centre suggested that the required information should be sought from the Chairman of the Management Committee. Unfortunately for the Panel, the Chairman's position had been made plain already in a letter dated 6 May, and delivered by his wife on the following day to the Office of the Assistant Director Care Services. In his reply, the Chairman of the Management Committee asked the now familiar question - under what statutory power was the Council conducting its inquiry?

Essentially, the Registered Homes Act 1984 gave the Borough little leverage over the Home. The only power the Borough had was threat of closure. In the absence of any offer of financial or other material help, it was unlikely that the power to delay closure could achieve little more than delay the closure of the Charity or the removal of the Home to cheaper premises. In view of the dearth of other suitable premises in the Borough removal to another local authority area was inevitable. In the case of a national charity, the Borough had no power to prevent such a move, despite a wish to retain the facility within its boundaries. Unless the Council had the will and the means to accommodate the residents of the Home there was no alternative to watching them being bundled into their coach and taken off to the Hotel.

NOTES

[1] Supplementary Benefit regulations for those in private and voluntary nursing and residential homes changed in 1983.

[2] A ceiling was placed on the amount DHSS was prepared to pay towards the costs of those on Supplementary Benefit in private and voluntary nursing and residential homes in September 1984.

[3] Centre for Policy on Aging, Home Life: a code of practice for Residential Care, 1984.

[4] For example, Jones, D. and Mayo, M., Community Work One, Routledge and Kegan Paul, 1974; and by the same authors, Community Work Two, Routledge and Kegan Paul, 1975.

[5] Sainsbury, S., Deaf Worlds.

[6] Ibid.

[7] Kramer, J. and Piachaud, D., 'The Micro-Economics of Old People's Homes', British Journal of Social Work, 12, 1982, pp. 171-187. Also, Sainsbury, S., op. cit.

8 The Home, the Hotel, and the Registered Homes Act 1984

As we have seen, the catalyst which brought about the removal of the elderly deaf residents from their Home in an inner London borough to a country hotel, three miles from a small market town in a county bordering Greater London, was the Registered Homes Act 1984. Yet, in many ways, the Act was utilised by both the Borough and the members of the Charity's Management Committee of Trustees in a manner which was largely unintended by those who framed the measure.

The Home and the Act, November 1984 to October 1985

The initial requirement for the re-registration of the Home in 1984 arose from the departure of the Matron who had held the Registration Certificate since 1978, and her replacement in July by the Director in Charge. In her report on the registration visit of November 7 1984, the Registration Officer for the Home used the new Registration Act to define the Home as ineligible for registration. Yet the Act was not due to come into force until 1 January 1985. Until that time, registration should have taken place under the Act of 1980. It seems clear that the new Act was used by the Director in Charge of the Home and the Registration Officer to bounce the Borough into acknowledging the Home's hopeless situation. It is odd, though consistent with the Borough's lack of policy towards residential care in the voluntary sector, that policy makers and management within the Borough had failed to appreciate that this was so. On the face of it, it may be considered extraordinary that the Borough's policy makers had not sought to devise a systematic response to such an important piece of legislation. However, the London boroughs had set up a panel to devise guidelines for registration under the Act which were intended to operate throughout the Greater London area to ensure a substantially systematic approach to private and voluntary homes throughout the region. That such guidance was necessary if standard criteria were to be applied within a local authority is clear from even a cursory reading of the Act and Regulations. [1]

The Regulations are discussed more fully later, but it is important to note that they abound with qualifying phrases such as 'as is reasonable', 'adequate to the well being of residents', and 'as far as is practicable', which themselves require definition if the Act is to be applied in a standard manner. Indeed, it is the lack of definition of such qualifying terms as applied to the Regulations concerning personal space for residents and the degree to which residents should be involved with fire drill which substantially diminishes the force of the criticism mounted by the Registration Officer of the six bedded rooms and the inability of residents to participate in fire drill because of the hazards of the building for the frail elderly. Had the Social Services Department's Directorate been aware of the degree to which the Regulations were open to interpretation on such issues, it is unlikely that the Registration Officer and Acting Director would have been able to create the atmosphere of crisis within the Social Services Department with regard to the Home's future.

However, if the absence of a policy with regard to the Act is to be explained by the delay in the publication of the London Guidelines until May 1985, and therefore as a conscious policy in its own right, it might be expected that the Borough's Social Services Department would not have become entangled prematurely in the application of the Act. Still less would the Social Services Directorate have accepted the assessment of the Home produced by the Registration Officer according to the Act's Regulations. Therefore it must be assumed that the Directorate had no policy of awaiting the Guidelines, accepted the Registration Officer's interpretation of the Act, and saw no reason to oppose her use of the Act. Indeed, it was reliance on her interpretation of the Act in the absence of any policy of its own regarding the Regulations, which enabled the Registration Officer to use the

Act as a threat to the future of the Home. Much of the discussion of a date for closure appears to have been spearheaded by the Registration Officer, a discussion with which the Directorate merely fell in, as it did with the assessment of the Home. In fact, the Social Services Directorate showed a marked reluctance to name a closure day, and especially so once health and safety standards had been met by improvements at the Home. Yet the threat of closure under the Act by the Directorate appears to have been used by the Management Committee to pressure residents and staff at the Home to move to the Hotel.

There were safeguards built into the Act which were never mentioned in connection with the Home's closure, presumably because closure was the overriding objective to the Management Committee. Furthermore, there was little attempt on the part of the Management Committee to ascertain, in accordance with the provisions of the new legislation, the wishes and feelings of residents on the matter of the move, and to give 'due consideration' to them, which would have been appropriate once health and safety standards had been met by improvements at the Home. In fact, it is evident that residents had two courses open to them, even though their opposition to the move was evident from the outset - to move to the Hotel together, or leave their group for their local authority of origin. Nor, it seems clear, did the Management Committee provide the residents in writing with the name and address of the Registration Authority, to which, under the Act, they had the right to make a complaint directly or through others acting on their behalf. There were other departures from the requirements of the new Act as well. For example, there is considerable evidence that the Management Committee systematically deprived the Borough of information, which the Social Services Department regarded as crucial, in direct contravention of the Act's requirement that the registration authority be given as much information as is reasonably required. Still less was there any attempt to abide by the London guidelines [2] which stressed the importance of not removing people from their own localities: most of the residents had been living in the Home for so long that they regarded its neighbourhood as their own locality, and such community ties as they had were there.

It seems clear, therefore, that the new Act was not applied systematically to the Home, but partially, and in such a way that the standards which it was assumed to prescribe were used to destroy the possibility of the Home's continued existence. Yet this destruction could only be achieved in the absence of a clear policy with respect to the Act on the part of the Borough's Social Services Department.

Yet even the physical standards required under the Act are open to wide interpretation, and in many cases could not be used in themselves as criteria according to which the acceptability of standards prevailing at the Home could be judged. For example, accommodation for each resident during the day and the night is required to be 'reasonable'; furniture, bedding, curtains and floor coverings must be 'adequate and suitable'; there must be a 'sufficient number' of WCs, washbasins, baths and showers with hot and cold water; light heating and ventilation must be 'adequate'; kitchen equipment, crockery, and cutlery are required to be 'sufficient and suitable'; 'adequate' facilities for the preparation and storage of food must be provided, while 'adequate' facilities for residents to prepare their own food and refreshment are to be made available 'so far as it is reasonable and practicable in the circumstances'.

In fact the Regulations reflect an attempt to detail good practice without jeopardising mediocre homes by the insistence on absolute standards. As such, not only are specific physical facilities such as kitchen equipment, toilet and washing facilities, carpets, curtains and so on, itemised, but so are aspects of care practice which have gained support as being 'progressive' because they maximise choice, privacy and personal space for residents as well as other conditions which help to recreate 'normality' for those in residential homes. An obvious example, is the emphasis placed by the Regulations on the necessity for the residents of homes to be able to maintain contact with relatives and others to whom they are close. Thus those in charge of homes are required to guarantee access to the public telephone system, and, 'as is reasonable and practicable' in the circumstances, to arrange for residents to communicate in private by post or telephone. Furthermore, facilities must be provided for visits by the relatives or friends of residents, as well as facilities for residents, if they wish to do so, to communicate privately with visitors, while visiting times must be displayed and information regarding visiting times must be made available to anyone who requires it. Another example is that residents should be encouraged 'to pursue existing interests or acquire new ones' and to 'participate in' policy making regarding the home and the way in which it is run, though such practices cannot be used as a substitute for the maintenance of proper staffing and standards.

Many such regulations are hedged about by qualification

which may allow a home to excuse its failure to comply with a particular requirement. However, there are regulations to which no such qualification is attached. These include procedures regarding the notification of the registration authority of the death of a resident, and the absence of the person in charge; the notification of the next of kin of the termination of a resident's accommodation in a home; the provision of information to residents regarding the method of making complaints about the home; and the right of access for the inspection of homes by the registration authority and representatives of the Secretary of State.

Perhaps surprisingly, staffing levels, and the quality of training of staff employed are not the subject of precise standards laid down in the regulations. It may be objected that it would be unusual for legislation and associated regulations in the field of the personal social services to be specific about either the quantity or the quality of staff. Yet it must be remembered that the Children's Act 1948 was specific about both the type and the training of those who were to man the new children's services. More recently, the government has attempted to regulate to ensure that only social workers who are specially trained for the purpose may be engaged in the process of depriving mentally ill people of their liberty. [3] In the case of the Registered Homes Act, however, the regulations are content to stipulate merely the necessity for 'suitably qualified staff ... in numbers adequate to the well-being of residents'.

The regulations were closely modelled on a document produced for the DHSS by the Centre for Policy on Aging in 1984. [4] The document had as its objective an attempt to provide guidance for practice in residential homes, and was based on the concensus on good practice which has emerged from the critique of residential care which received widespread approval in the 1960s. Hence the emphasis placed on 'integration' into the community rather than segregation from it; and the attempt to create 'normality' by encouraging elderly people to participate in the organisation of the home, and to maintain as far as possible, the activities which are customary in private households by seeking to enable residents to do their own laundry and make snacks for themselves; and the maintenance of links with the past by ensuring facilities which encourage visits to the homes from the relatives and friends of residents. Similarly, there is an emphasis on the importance of providing private space in which each resident may seek to recreate the atmosphere of a private household. It is interesting to note that, as was the case in the anti-institutional literature on which it was based, on the question of participation in household chores, there is no mention in the document of role differences as between men and women among the elderly population, nor is there any consideration of the possibility that some elderly people may not wish to continue to look after themselves, regardless of their degree of frailty.

Normatively prescribed criteria according to which 'normality' might be achieved, have been lifted uncritically from the academic literature on institutions, and built into legislation. Perhaps it is fortunate for some elderly people that many regulations <u>are</u> hedged about with qualifications. It is astonishing that assumptions regarding the 'normal' lives of elderly people in private households which were based on an idealised pattern of living described in the 1950s should continue to exercise such influence on policy makers and academics alike.

What is interesting is the failure to compare systematically requirements for institutions with the generality of the provision available in private households, the generally accepted most desirable setting for life at any age. When, in <u>The Registered Homes Act 1984: Guidance for Registration</u>, produced for the London boroughs in May 1985, the direct comparison is made between the two settings, it is assumed that private households provide a pattern for upholding 'fundamental rights to dignity, self determination and individuality' and a 'full and active life as ... physical and mental condition permit'. Furthermore, 'the manner and circumstances in which they (the residents) live should as far as is possible, equate to the normal domestic practice of those who continue to live in the community'. Even a cursory review of the conditions of those who are dependent while living in private households would query the degree to which 'self determination' is the norm: it is customary for domiciliary services whether provided by the formal or informal network, to be made available in the time and manner convenient to the giver rather than the recipient. Similar criticism may be made about assumptions concerning personal space, especially where elderly people live with relatives, and the privacy available to <u>anyone</u> who is dependent on another for personal help.

In the advice given to the London boroughs on the application of the Act, the regulations are elaborated upon, to provide a blue print for good practice. Thus the regulation requiring adequate space for each resident during the day and at night is translated into a specific requirement for single, or at most two-bedded rooms. Indeed, throughout, there is a tendency to define the regulations in optimum terms. But it is important to note that it is not expected that all existing registered establishments will be able to reach such levels of provision in the short term: it is envisaged that the registration authority will adopt an interventionist approach to homes which have difficulty in meeting regulations, by encouraging a gradual improvement in the standard of their facilities and care practices. That being so, it is difficult to understand why, once the health and safety regulations had been satisfied, record keeping improved, and the management of the Home raised to acceptable levels - as was claimed by the Management Committee in the Charity's Report for 1984/5, the Home could not have continued in the existing premises. Certainly, the new Registration Act, which had been used to precipitate the crisis, posed no immediate threat to the Home's continued existence.

The Hotel

However, as we have seen, by the early summer of 1985, the rationale for the move from the Home to the Hotel had shifted from the immediate repercussions of the Act to the necessity to make a large profit on the sale of the old property and the purchase of the new to ensure the availability of funds which would be adequate to the purchase of premises which fully accorded with the highest standards required by modern expectations of residential care, and to enable the Charity to improve its financial viability by increasing the number of residents.

Under the new Registration Act, the Registration Authority has to approve new premises before they can be used for residential accommodation. It seems clear from the records that the Hotel was purchased by the Management Committee before the acquisition of such authorisation, and that the New Authority was prepared to refuse to sanction the use of the Hotel for this purpose, if the Borough had been prepared to accept the consequences. As we know, the Borough was never prepared to be committed to the provision of material resources to ensure the continuation of the Home. When a visit was made subsequently to the Hotel in November 1986, by the Borough's Senior Social Worker (Deaf) and the Panel of Inquiry's outside Assessor, the New Authority's Registration Officer made it plain that she would never have agreed to the conversion of the Hotel to a residential Home: its remote rural situation made it impossible for residents to go out on their own or integrate easily into the neighbourhood, while there must be doubt that however extensive the adaptations undertaken, a hotel could not be made to feel like a home. However, even she had to admit that the Management Committee had achieved a remarkable conversion.

Within the hotel, the elderly deaf residents now lived in exceptionally comfortable surroundings. All the rooms and passages were well carpeted and the whole building was comfortably warm. The day rooms had been well adapted: neither the dining room nor the sitting rooms appeared to be those of an institution or an hotel. There were plenty of warm and comfortable arm chairs in the sitting rooms, and the residents were cosily sitting around knitting, watching television, and chatting. In terms of personal space, residents were well catered for, most in single bedrooms, the rest being in twin-bedded rooms. Staff reported that where sharing took place, they ensured that only those who were compatible were put together in a bedroom. All but one of the bedrooms had substantial wardrobes (one resident had to make do with a curtained rail) and they were all well furnished with chests of drawers and bedside tables. In many rooms, a few decorative personal possessions, such as souvenir dolls, were left on dressing tables and chairs. Residents were allowed to have televisions in their rooms, but none had shown any disposition to do so - they preferred to be together downstairs. All rooms had their own washing facilities, and almost all had their own bath or shower and WC.

An easy relationship could be observed to exist between staff and residents. Residents felt free to make themselves tea in addition to that which was generally available. One resident was having her hair washed and set. Everyone appeared to be at ease. Staffing levels were good, and staff commitment to the Hotel high. All members of staff had attended short sign language courses and could communicate with residents at a basic level. And at least as important, staff appeared to be willing to spend time to engage in communication with residents. Some members of staff had made arrangements to attend courses in geriatrics. There was evidence to suggest that staff were able to cope well with death among the residents. Two residents had been nursed in the final stages of terminal illness at the Hotel, which was equipped with adequate resources for carrying out that task.

All residents received their statutory allowance, and they all spent it, usually in the nearby town. Whenever members of staff went into town, they usually took a resident with them. Furthermore, there were regular group outings in the minibus: apart from their continued attendance at the Day Centre in the Borough to maintain the links they had established at the Home, they also visited other centres with a deaf population nearer the Hotel, and themselves received such groups as visitors.

The families of residents continued to visit the Hotel and treat it as an extension of their own homes. At the Open Day held to mark the first anniversary of the Hotel as a residential home for deaf women, the relatives of the two residents who had died in the course of that year, came to help, and continued to return to visit other residents whom they had come to regard as part of their own family. The Open Day itself indicated from the amount of local support given to it, that despite an unforseen clash with a similar occasion held that day by another, well established local voluntary organisation, the Hotel had quickly become a focus of local interest, and could well become a recognised part of the local community.

It was clear that the residents at the Hotel were operating as an interdependent community. When issues arose for discussion about the day to day running of the Hotel, collective decisions were taken and presented to the staff. To a considerable extent, the staff were now part of that community.

In general then, a considerable balancing act had been achieved. Within the institutional framework of the provision of shelter, warmth and good food, a considerable degree of comfort had been established both by the availability of good and appropriate furnishings, and staff capable of and willing to engage in conversation with residents; in addition, however, a reasonable degree of privacy was assured, and choice preserved, partly by the availability of private space, but also by the freedom to make tea, help in decision making within the home, and exercise such economic decisions as are possible within the limits of the statutory allowance. Furthermore, 'integration' into 'normal' life was pursued by successfully encouraging the continued interest of relatives in the Hotel's residents, and, increasingly, of those living in the neighbourhood, as well as by fostering contact with other groups of deaf people. Yet the residents remained in their traditional inter-dependent and tightly knit community. The ideal before which everyone currently interested in social policy regularly makes obeisance, and which is held to be the hall-mark of life outside institutions, but which generally, when sought, proves to be elusive or non-existent, triumphantly flourishes within this particular institution.

Yet there were causes for concern. There appeared to be little evidence that the New Registration Authority was able to place specialist skills in deaf welfare at the service of the Hotel. Indeed, the Registration Officer made it clear that she had no specialist knowledge in this area. It was interesting to have a clear example of the way in which lack of specialist knowledge could lead to a total misunderstanding of a situation. The Registration Officer declared openly that she was not in favour of residential care and argued that however well adapted an establishment was, it nevertheless retained the appearance and atmosphere of an institution. As an example, she drew attention to the arrangement of the armchairs in the otherwise well adapted sitting rooms - she wished they were not set out in a circle around the television. A member of staff replied that residents were responsible for the arrangement. Although she admitted this point, the Registration Officer remained unhappy. It took the Borough's Senior Social Worker (Deaf) to explain that the circle of chairs ensured that everyone could see the television, and, much more important, that everyone could see everyone else signing.

The community within the Hotel, like most successful communities, has developed not by design, but out of necessity, and, to some extent, adversity. It is based primarily on a common language, the shared experience of communication difficulties with the hearing, and long acquaintance - all of which are the supports of the cohesiveness of the deaf community outside institutions. It is ironic that when faced with the existence of a community, at least some of those who claim it as an ideal should seek its destruction. There have always been those who have disapproved of the 'segregated' deaf community, and have sought to 'integrate' deaf people into the hearing world where a sense of community is considerably less marked. So it is in the case of the Hotel. The threat to the residents' community comes from two main directions - the New Registration Authority, and the Charity's Management Committee. Perhaps the most obvious threat comes from the interaction of these two pressures with a third, namely time. Over many years death has caused the contraction of the community of deaf residents. It was the failure of the Home to counteract the effect of death on the community by attracting new residents which originally aroused the concern of the Management Committee for the viability of the Charity in the mid-1970s. Since moving to the Hotel, a further two residents have died. At the time of the visit, there was the prospect of one new permanent resident. But the shortfall in residents was being met with two short stay residents. A switch of emphasis to short stay temporary accommodation would have the blessing of many interested in the personal social services. In the general and widely applauded denigration of long term institutional care, an acceptable role for residential care has been discerned in the provision of short term rehabilitative care even for the elderly. Such a course for the Hotel, as a way out of the Management Committee's difficulties in attracting new residents, would probably have considerable support locally. The New Registration Authority has adopted an anti-institutional policy, and goes to considerable lengths to avoid admission into residential care even of those who wish to enter a home. [5]

Indeed, the Registration Officer betrayed her support for this approach when she indicated that homes 'should improve people so that they can leave'. However, both she and the Hotel staff recognised the difficulties involved in mixing temporary with permanent residents. It was apparent on the day of the visit that the two temporary residents remained apart from the others. While the group should be able to absorb new long-term residents - it must have done so successfully in the past - there is little doubt that short term residents have neither the time to establish relationships with the group nor the commitment to do so.

Furthermore, the overall social policy objective of ensuring a 'normal home life' for everyone, by emphasising the superiority and goal, of life and care in private households for those who are dependent is based on the assumption that such households are 'integrated' into the 'community'. As such, it is a policy which denies the possibility of the creation of a sense of community within an institutional setting, or, when faced with such a community, regards it as a regrettable aberration, because it subsumes individual autonomy. Thus, the Registration Officer considered it to be wrong that deaf residents should reach collective decisions, and present them collectively. It is a point of view which underscores the highly individualised styles of living prevalent in our society, while paying lip service to notions of community or defining community as no more than the aggregate of highly autonomous individualised lives.

Symptomatic of this point of view was the desire of the Registration Officer to introduce the key worker system into the Hotel, so that each resident would have an individual to whom they could 'relate'. This was a notion which at one and the same time underscored the importance of highly individualised rather than inter-dependent living, and emphasised the rehabilitative view of residential care. Moreover, the introduction of the key worker system could well undermine the role of the Hotel as a home.

Indeed, the failure to perceive the role of the Hotel as the home for a collection of elderly deaf women was implicit in the insistence of the Registration Officer (in quoting her Director of Social Services) on talking about the Hotel as a 'facility'. The term emerged in the course of a discussion regarding the use of a long day room, one side of which almost entirely consisted of windows. Without the leather benches arranged along the windows, it could have had the appearance of a grand conservatory. This was the only room below the second floor not to have been refurbished or adapted in any way, and at least part of the reason for this was the absence of any firm decision as to its use. At the time it was used only for functions involving large numbers of people - it had proved to be handy during the Open Day - and as the place in which the hair dresser set the residents' hair. The Director of Social Services was reported as favouring its use for activities engaged in by groups from outside the Hotel, preferably groups of people not associated with the deaf world. One suggestion was that the room could be used as a Day Centre, perhaps for the physically handicapped: such a proposal, it was argued, should involve consulting the deaf residents to discover, not whether they would approve of such a development in their home, but whether they wished it to be part of their home, or a separate entity. [6]

It was clear that for a local authority which regarded residential care as an option to be avoided at all costs, the barriers to conceeding the Hotel to be home for a collection deaf women were considerable. Those barriers have their origin in the 1960s, when misunderstandings arose concerning the use of the terms 'community' and 'integration'. Community studies based on an anthropological approach focussed on interconnectedness in neighbourhood relationships, and discovered in such communities considerable interdependence. [7] Thus, the idea of communities of interconnectedness in neighbourhoods, which were also interdependent, developed. However, it was clear from such studies, that interdependence was strongly associated with local kinship ties, within which women played a dominant role. Indeed, later studies undertaken to explore the impact of the destruction of traditional neighbourhoods on interconnected communities stressed the survival of the interdependent kinship network, especially the crucial mother-daughter relationship, and the importance of the female members of the family in undertaking the caring role, despite geographic mobility and the consequent dispersal of the kinship network. [8]

Thus mobility destroyed interdependence based on neighbourhood, but not necessarily interconnectedness. Indeed, subsequent studies of dependent groups such as mentally and physically handicapped people, undertaken in the 1960s and 1970s, showed, as had earlier studies of elderly people living at home, that care is very much a private family affair. [9] The most that can be expected of interconnection with those other than kin in a neighbourhood, is help on an ad hoc basis, which commits no one to sustained intervention in a household. [10] Indeed, so private is care, that its provision is usually restricted to relatives within the household of the dependent person, or, where these do not exist, to one or two, usually female relatives deemed to be appropriate to the task, and convenient because of their geographical proximity to the dependent person.

The difficulty emerged when government was forced to abandon its definition of 'community care' as non-hospital care, that is, any care, residential or domiciliary, paid for out of local government resources, in favour of non-residential care, by social scientists who were influential in setting the social policy agenda during the 1960s. The consequent confusion emerges clearly in the pages of the Last Refuge, where the idea of the right of everyone to a normal life is expounded, and normality identified with the interdependence within private households, between the generations of members of individual families. The problem was, however, that the book had shown that elderly people in residential care were there precisely because they lacked appropriate, particularly female, relatives. In so far as this problem was addressed, it was assumed that surrogate relatives in the shape of domiciliary services and neighbours trained for the purpose and organised by social workers would effectively undertake 'community care'. However, none of the post war investigations of communities and care suggested that neighbours were accustomed to such a role. Recent research has suggested that there may well have been some interdependence as well as interconnectedness among neighbours who were not kin in some working class localities in the past, which was generated by the commonly experienced disasters of poverty and long term unemployment. [11] But there appears to be little evidence to suggest that even where neighbourhoods are brought together by shared disaster the privacy within which the systematic interdependence required by care commonly prevails is often breached.

Thus the assumption that the 'community' will respond to dependent people is based on a misapprehension about the nature of community, interconnectedness, and interdependence in our society. People are recognised as being in 'the community' if they adopt the social norms of interdependence within the privacy of the household and the family, whilst enjoying limited interconnectedness with non-kinship groups in the neighbourhood and beyond. Indeed, groups which display interdependence outside the kinship network may be regarded as aberrant - for example, members of the deaf community, among whom there is considerable interdependence for acquiring information about the hearing community, certain religious sects, and some minority ethnic groups, are regarded by many with suspicion, because their members do not adopt the highly individualised style of living, based on the family within the private household, which alone is considered to be normal. Thus policy, both national and local together with their underlying theories and general assumptions about what is appropriate in our society, posed a threat to the long-established interdependent community of mainly elderly deaf women, which now occupied the Hotel.

In addition, however, further threats were posed by the difficulties and behaviour of the Charity's Management Committee. Because the Hotel was purchased in haste, and, in its final stages the transaction was undertaken in some secrecy, the property was never fully investigated in partnership with the Registration Authority before purchase, to establish the full extent of the adaptations required. The Management Committee considered that the sale of the Home was imperative because the long-term financial viability of the Charity was dependent upon attracting and accommodating a larger number of residents. The accommodation for such an expansion was now available on the top floor of the Hotel, but could not be used until a lift had been installed. However, the adaptations required by the New Registration Authority under the Registered Homes Act 1984, were becoming so costly, that despite the large profit made on the sale of the Home, the Management Committee were finding it difficult to raise the £40,000 which, it was estimated, the lift installation and other adaptations were likely to cost. Uncertainty as to the probable position of the lift in part explained the failure to adapt the long lounge. Thus in certain respects, the members of the Management Committee had returned to the position they were in with the Home: to be financially viable in the long-term they had to attract and accommodate more residents, but to do this required an outlay of money which they did not have. As a consequence, a major fundraising programme was to be embarked upon, for which the Hotel's Director was to be given a large measure of responsibility. The Registration Officer expressed doubts about the wisdom of requiring the Director both to retain full responsibility for the day to day management of the Hotel and to undertake a substantial fundraising role: was such a combination usual, she wondered, in homes for the deaf? It must be admitted, of course, that it is not usual. While persons in charge of homes for the deaf normallly have responsibility for managing the budget, and perhaps raising small sums of money through sales of work, open days and so on, in general, they are not required to play a major part in raising funds for their charities. [12] It is interesting to speculate as to why the Management Committee were now so confident of their capacity to raise money for the

Charity, when they had been so convinced that nothing of the sort could be done for the Home, that no one was likely to give worthwhile amounts of money for residential accommodation, that residential homes all over the country were experiencing similar financial difficulties, and that the considerable efforts which they had already made in this respect had had only a derisory response. After all, it was for this reason that profit from the sale of property was seen as the only solution to the Charity's financial difficulties.

Other difficulties attached to the behaviour of members of the Management Committee. For example, although up to the time of the visit, no member of the Management Committee had any specialist knowledge about deaf people and the deaf community, they were accustomed to issue directives on the way in which the Hotel was to be run. Hotel staff, most of whom had attended at least a brief course in sign language, considered that they now understood a little about deafness in general, knew well their deaf residents in particular, and resented having to carry out commands with which they often disagreed, but about which there was no opportunity for discussion. Furthermore, not only were staff excluded from the monthly meeting between the Hotel's Director, the residents and the Management Committee held in accordance with the Registered Homes Act 1984, they were not involved in setting the agenda for discussion at the meeting, nor were their views sought and represented there. Of course, it may be argued that such meetings have been so organised precisely to protect the interests of residents, to allow them to express views free from the pressure exerted by the presence of those who care for them on a daily basis. But while that may be the case, it would seem to be wise, especially in view of the degree to which staff had become part of the Hotel's community, and the energy with which they sought to acquire appropriate expertise in their field of care, that an effective avenue should have been provided by which their views could be transmitted to the Management Committee.

In conclusion, then, it seems clear on the basis of observation, that the residents of the Hotel now enjoyed a high standard of living in surroundings of considerable comfort, cared for by understanding and committed staff, albeit in a rather isolated, rural setting, and removed from their original neighbourhood contacts, though some of these were maintained by visits by minibus to their old Day Centre in the Borough. Their small interdependent community remained unimpaired. But the tranquility of their new home was threatened by the possible introduction of a substantial element of short term care to the Hotel, the development of part of the Hotel as a facility for outside groups, who would probably not include deaf people, the emphasis of the New Registration Authority on rehabilitation and the desirability of individualised as opposed to communal living, and the behaviour of members of the Management Committee who had failed once more to ensure the financial viability of the Charity, and who offend staff, whose views are not taken into account when decisions are made.

NOTES

[1] Regulations under Registered Homes Act 1984, Statutory Instrument No. 1345, 1984.

[2] The Registered Homes Act 1984: Guidance for Registration, May 1985, first edition.

[3] Mental Health Act 1983.

[4] Centre for Policy on Aging, op. cit.

[5] For a reflection of attitudes on residential care which are currently popular, see for example, Booth, T., Home Truths - Old People's Homes and the Outcome of Care, Gower, 1985; Clough, R., Residential Social Work, Macmillan, 1982; and Clough, R., Beyond Barclay: the future of residential care, Social Care Association, 1981.

[6] Willmott, P. and Young, M., Family and Kinship in East London, Routledge and Kegan Paul, 1957; Wilmott, P. and Young, M., Family and Class in a London Suburb, Routledge and Kegan Paul, 1960; Townsend, P., The Family Life of Old People.

[7] Rosser, C. and Harris, C., The Family and Social Change, Routledge and Kegan Paul, 1965.

[8] Bayley, M., Mental Handicap and Community Care, Routledge and Kegan Paul, 1973; also, Sainsbury, S., Registered as Disabled.

[9] Sainsbury, S., ibid.; also, Sainsbury, S., Disability and Social Policy, forthcoming.

[10] Abrams, P., 'Realities of Neighbourhood Care', Policy and Politics, vol. 12, no. 4, 1984.

[11] Sainsbury, S., Deaf Worlds.

9 Conclusions

It is salutary to remember who was meant to benefit from the agitation and conflict described here. The purpose of those on all sides - the Management Committee of the Charity, elected members of the Borough Council, Officers of the Social Services Department, and members of interested local community groups - was to promote the welfare of a group of profoundly, prelingually elderly deaf women for whom residential accommodation was provided by the Charity. Throughout the period covered by the study, no one involved with the Home would have dissented from the analysis of its residents' situation presented by the Social Services Department in a background information paper dated 18 September 1985, and drawn up for the benefit of the Panel of Inquiry:

> The clients at the ... Home ... are all very vulnerable women. Most of them are elderly and have been living in (the Borough) for a very long time and ... (the Borough) is, in fact, their home. None of them can communicate coherently with the hearing officers and they have very little power of control over their own lives.
>
> Consequently their inability to represent their own interests, to express their feelings and opinions means that they will have less opportunity to protect their

interests. In short, they cannot fully participate in any decision making process which has implications for their welfare. It is therefore right for the Department of Social Services to ensure, through its professionals, that the long term interests of all the residents are secured.

It has been the purpose of this study to consider why, when there was general agreement as to the accuracy of the Department's analysis, and in the face of widespread community and Council opposition, the women were removed against their will from accommodation and an inner city locality which most of them had regarded as home for more than two decades, to a country hotel in another county, and three miles from the nearest town. When the removal to the Hotel had taken place, the Chairman of the local Voluntary Association for the Elderly asked the Assistant Director Care Services why the Local Authority did not pursue its duty with more vigour and use its powers to investigate the well being of residents and the standards of management at the Home?

The answer to these questions has been found in the changes in the focus of policy within the personal social services and their administrative structure which took place in the early 1970s. Since the nineteenth century, many residential homes in the voluntary sector have become accustomed to depend indirectly upon public funding through maintenance fees paid by public bodies which sponsor residents in the homes. With the years, the importance of such funding to charities providing residential accommodation has increased dramatically, and the policy of the last seven years, with its emphasis on the role of Social Services Departments as assessors for, rather than providers of services, has served to accentuate such dependence still further, yet public control over such charitable endeavours is weak. The National Assistance Act 1948, which placed the duty for registering voluntary and private homes on local authorities, was open to a laissez faire interpretation, and a patchwork of widely differing responses to it grew up. Some homes were never registered, others were visited only once for registration purposes, still others were inspected regularly once a year or even more often. The other method of exerting influence, if not control, over the management of a voluntary home was to rely on informal links established by a member of the council or one of its senior officers acquiring a seat on the management committee. Yet despite the weakness of the mechanisms by which influence could be exerted, the present study indicates that not only was a measure of control possible, it could happen even where the client group concerned, for reasons of tradition and problems of communication was unlikely to attract the attention of local authority policy makers and service providers. However, the prerequisites for such practice emerged as threefold. First, there had to be a clear departmental policy which interpreted the general social policy goals of 'promotional welfare' to include active intervention to determine the standard of voluntary residential care; second, a determination was required that the mechanism for achieving such a policy was that the duty to visit for registration purposes should be undertaken regularly and frequently; and finally, residents should be visited regularly and care staff supported by a specialist worker directly responsible to the chief officer in charge of the policy. It is clear that during the years 1965-1972 when such a system operated in the Borough, a steady and significant improvement in the management of the Home was maintained.

The changes introduced in 1972 as a result of the Local Authority Social Services Act 1970, ensured that with the amalgamation of the services of the welfare and children's departments and many of those of the health departments into a single social services department, and the emphasis placed on genericism, the source of growing specialist skills - parochial concern with 'my deaf' - was largely obliterated. In the unified department, the deaf slipped even further from the centre of directorial preoccupation, which was increasingly dominated by the problem of children, and the claims of community pressure groups. Even a concern for residential care appeared less pressing as the campaign against institutional care became increasingly fashionable and acceptable. Responsibility for maintaining contact with the Home was devolved to an Area Office. There was no follow through from the directorate, no policy of utilising the registration process to promote welfare within the Home, and there was and never had been, an alternative system of exerting influence through the informal links established by elected members, their wives, or officers of the council sitting on the Management Committee. As a consequence, between 1973 and 1984, there was only one Registration Visit - that of 1978. Moreover, there is clear evidence that within a few years of the end of the Borough's policy of interventionist promotional welfare, the Charity began to experience considerable difficulties: its Trustees required a loan from the Council to carry out essential structural repairs and alterations, and they asked for the Director's help in determining the Charity's future role. In both instances the response from the Borough was positive, but it is clear that each request was seen as originating in a discreet problem, and the troubles of the Home were not regarded as having policy implications for the Department.

In 1984, at the end of this period of benign neglect, the day to day management of the Home became so difficult that an Acting Director had to be brought in from a national voluntary association for the deaf, and the Management Committee decided to wind up the Charity. That the welfare of the Charity's existing beneficiaries was not the concern of the Charity Commissioners now became apparent. Their duty was to ensure the continued existence of the Charity for as long as there were beneficiaries. Therefore, the closure of the Charity was prevented, and a policy of selling the existing Home to purchase cheaper accommodation which was to be refurbished to registerable standards with the profits of the sale, was devised. As this was a national Charity, the location of the new accommodation did not matter.

By the time that the Social Services Department decided to implement the Registered Homes Act 1984, and reverse its policy, now more than a decade old, of somnolent non-intervention, a clear policy had been devised for the Home by its Management Committee, but no comparable thought had been given by the Local Authority to the policy implications of the Act in general, or the consequences of its application to this particular Home. The Registration Officer applied the new assessment criteria to the Home, and saw the Home and its problems through the eyes of its Acting Director, and under the influence of policies already established by the Management Committee, and apparently unsullied by the views of the social workers at the local Area Officer who appear to have remained untroubled by the Home's standards of care. The Directorate appear to have accepted the judgement of the Registration Officer without question, and in the absence of any pre-existing policy for responding to the implications of that judgement, were forced to evolve a policy as the crisis developed.

An early decision was taken that the women should be kept together, but beyond that, at the outset, the policy of the Management Committee was accepted without question. However, it soon became clear that the preferred option of the Local Authority was to delay the Prohibition Order in the hope that the Charity would find the money to carry out the necessary works: only in the event of the failure to find the cash would the sale of the Home be regarded as acceptable. Even then, the assumption appeared to be that alternative accommodation would be found within the borough. When the dearth of suitable accommodation within the Borough became clear, and the Charity's resources stretched only to bringing the Home up to Health and Safety, not Registration standards - the dormitories remained a stumbling block - was the determination to sell and purchase elsewhere made clear. The Borough's response was to set up an investigation of the Charity. A certain langour which had characterised the Borough's approach to the Charity since the Registration Visit, appeared to continue even now. It is difficult to refute the position of the Chairman of the local Voluntary Association for the Elderly, in his letter to the Assistant Director Care Services on 15 November 1985, in which he asked if it had been the intention that if the Local Authority had dragged its heels, the problem would go away, and his observation that there had been a lot of activity but little action.

However, it would be unwise to minimise the difficulties of the Local Authority. The past had ensured that the Social Services Directorate had to make policy on its feet, and as a consequence, it was inevitable that there was a tendency to respond to events rather than take the initiative. Furthermore, the only alternative to closure or sale, once the Management Committee's view of the Charity's position was accepted, was for the Local Authority to offer material help - either by helping to raise the money to pay for all or a substantial part of the remaining works, or by issuing an injunction to prevent the move and taking responsibility for the residents. It was the decision that it could not commit resources which reduced the Local Authority to impotence. [1] The Registered Homes Act 1984, though requiring annual registration visits, is no more helpful than the National Assistance Act 1948 in determining how a Local Authority should respond to low standards. It remains the case that unless a voluntary organisation has both the will and the funds to bring an establishment up to standard, the Local Authority may lose the use of the facility through closure; sale and removal to ensure a Charity's continuance may be detrimental to the interests of a home's residents. Yet the only alternative may be direct provision by the local authority itself - a curious irony in view of the government's intention in passing the 1984 Act to provide greater control over, and therefore render more acceptable, voluntary rather than local authority provision.

In the course of the present study, the problem of that other traditional means of influencing the management of voluntary homes - the acquisition of places on the management committee by councillors, their wives, or council officers, emerged as the crisis developed. Such informal methods of influence never seem to have been part of the Borough's policy towards the Home, and when the Home's Management Committee on the advice of the Charity Commissioners, suggested to the local authority the cooption of knowledgeable councillors and officers, there appears to have been no response. Therefore the Management Committee sought such links unofficially, and those coopted were subsequently elected onto the Management Committee. Another, even more tenuous link between Home and Borough was provided by the Home's Registration Officer who was also the wife of the Chairman of the Management Committee. Even though such links were unofficial, it might have been expected that officers, who in their professional lives implemented Borough policy, would be likely to extend that policy's influence over the Home and its management. Unfortunately, other than the stipulation that the residents should be kept together, there was no clear policy formulated by the Borough with regard to the Home. It may well not have been obvious that there was a divergence of interest between Home and Borough until the Home's Management Committee had become committed to sale and repurchase, even if the new premises could be found only outside the Borough. After all, sale had been the policy for the Home since the early Autumn of 1984: the policy became a problem for the Local Authority only when it was pursued after it became clear that no suitable premises were available within the Borough. The desirability of keeping the residents within the locality then became an overt plank of policy. As a letter from the Chairman of the local Voluntary Association for the Elderly pointed out on 16 August 1985, it had to be admitted that the Management Committee had inherited a very difficult problem, but the policy of sale was wrong. It seems probable that had a policy of open discussion with community and council developed, rather than one of stealth and sale, the pressure on the Council and other bodies to produce resources might have been sufficient to obviate the sale.

However, removal appears to have been embarked upon without consultation with relatives, and against the wishes of residents, the Council and many local voluntary community groups. Furthermore, the actual date of removal was deliberately shrouded with mystery and kept from many relatives as well as the Council. While it is true that this was not the first time that a home for deaf people had been closed and the residents moved elsewhere, precedent does not necessarily justify such action, and what appears to have been without precedent was the manner of the removal. The isolation of deaf people from the hearing community appears to have been exploited to further policy. As the Director of Social Services informed the Chairman of the local Voluntary Association for the Elderly, no deadline was attached to the works required to bring the existing Home up to registration standard. Therefore, even in the very difficult circumstances which they inherited, it is hard to explain why Council officers on the Management Committee should have risked the degree of opprobrium which they must have known they would run in their place of employment, and which their professional experience and training would tell them would be disproportionate to any gains - whatever they were - which the continuation of the Committee's policy might promise. Perhaps they did not think through their position; perhaps their working relationships were so poor already that they did not care. Whatever the reason, their actions had serious consequences for 15 elderly deaf people and their relatives.

The risks which attach to reliance on informal links between local authority and voluntary home as a means of ensuring the council's influence with regard to standards of care and management have been revealed in the course of the present study. Such a control mechanism is satisfactory only when there is no divergence of interest between home and local authority, or when neither party is prepared to press its claims too closely. Public checks under registration provisions, at least for existing establishments, even when they utilise public funds extensively, albeit indirectly, are tenuous. The over-riding objective of charities, appears to be to survive for as long as there are beneficiaries. The Charity Commission is interested primarily in the viability of the charity: the welfare of current beneficiaries is by no means a major consideration.

Of course, excuses can be made, as they have been made here for the behaviour of both the Charity and the Borough, but neither emerge from the affair well. However, the persistence shown by a few voluntary groups, especially the local voluntary Association for the Elderly, in keeping the issue alive in a constructive way, is encouraging. Apart from that, admiration must be reserved for the dignity of the Home's residents and the integrity with which they perpetuated their small community of interdependent deaf people. It is sad to have to observe that the deaf community generally would find nothing surprising in being treated with such casual cruelty by the hearing.

Yet the present study raises an issue which is larger than the question of control over voluntary and private residential care institutions which are funded largely from the public purse. That issue concerns the control of the quality of care in <u>any</u> setting, whatever the provenance of its provision. We have been reminded recently that direct accountability to elected representatives does not obviate the necessity for concern in the arena of public provision. And disquiet about the nature and standard of care available in that pattern of perfection, the private household, provided by that guarantor of excellence, the family, is now being expressed openly. Wherever they are cared for, the dependent are vulnerable. The problem is to identify how an acceptable standard of care may be assured. The history of the relationship between the Home and the Borough shows that much may be achieved if a consciously determined policy is pursued systematically, and those who are expected to carry it out have the skills to do so, and are required to render an account of the performance of their duties.

NOTES

[1] Independent Review of Residential Care for the Elderly within the London Borough of Camden, 1987, unpublished report.

10 The regulation of voluntary and private homes

The study discussed here raises the general question of how far it is possible to regulate voluntary and private homes. That such regulation is necessary is clear not only from the evidence of the study, but from revelations by press and television of the appalling conditions and cruel treatment which are to be found in some private homes for the elderly. Even before the recent increase in the private provision of residential accommodation, television programmes about the abuse of elderly people in private residential homes endeavoured to create concern not only about the existence of abuse, but the rarity of local authority action and the ease with which the owner of a de-registered home was able to set up in business again under a new name. Prosecutions were rare and difficult to mount: witnesses tended to be low paid care or domestic assistants who felt obliged to give up their jobs before making accusations, while few other residential care workers were prepared to jeopardise their jobs at a time of high unemployment by offering corroborating evidence.

The purpose of the Registered Homes Act 1984 was to allay fears of the growth of such scandals with the rise of the number of residential homes outside the statutory sector, which was encouraged by the changes in the Supplementary Benefit regulations in 1983. Although the problem was one of long standing, it acquired political significance only in the context of the large scale dispersal of public funds to private and voluntary agencies unfettered by effective controls, at a time when local authority funds for residential care, as for all other services, were curtailed increasingly by government, in the first instance as part of an economic strategy, and later on political grounds.

Since the Act was passed, the major concern of local authorities has been to acquire adequate funding for the registration and inspection processes. They have pointed not only to the deployment of appropriate personnel as registration officers at a time when their powers to raise and spend money have been subject to increasing restriction. The solution proffered by government was not additional Exchequer contributions to local authorities, but arrangements whereby the costs of administering the Act could be recouped by local authority charges on voluntary and private homes for inspection and registration at levels set by the government. Not surprisingly, this led to tension between local authorities and DHSS regarding the adequacy of the prescribed levels. Belatedly, DHSS published the results of a survey which indicated that 'significant increases' were required if local authorities were to be fully reimbursed for the cost of adequate inspection and registration services. [1] Although the government agreed to large increases in both the registration and inspection fees (45 per cent and 73 per cent respectively) these were not regarded as satisfactory by local authorities. It seems clear that any level set by government is open to question, particularly with regard to inflation and the definition of an adequate service. The local authorities continue to argue that they should set their own rates for registering and inspecting the homes in their areas. [2]

Initially, little attention was paid to the efficacy of the Act as a means of regulation. Yet within two years of the Act coming into force, a Yorkshire television programme revealed abuse of residents in private homes for the elderly in Kent. The local authority reaction was to indicate the dilemma which faced the London Borough on which the present study focused, namely, that because they are short of resources, local authorities have no effective leverage. If a local authority confronts a recalcitrant management with the threat of closure, it must have the will and the resources to accept responsibility for the residents in the event of the threat being made effective. The response of the Kent social services department was coloured mainly by the lack of resources generally available to local authorities, but also by the county council's ideological commitment to non-institutional care and the private market. As a consequence, the County's practical measures have been restricted to improving its registration service. These included the employment of extra staff to enable more visits to be made: from 1988 all homes were to be visited four times a year, including two visits to be made unannounced, one of them at night. Part of the package of improvements, such as the appointment of a County Registration Officer, was said to predate the screening of the television programme. Other proposals for change were the computerisation of records, a computerised directory, discussions with the police about the possibility of seeing criminal records of prospective home owners, and a review of staff training in private homes to see where the social services department could help to improve training. [3]

Despite the focus of attention on the poor performance of some private homes in Kent, and the emphasis placed on the improvement of the registration and inspection process by the social services department as a means of improving standards in those homes, there was no evidence to suggest that the county's registration service could be regarded as below the generally accepted standard. Indeed, the Social Services Inspectorate, in a report on an investigation carried out before the screening of the programme, commended Kent's registration service, and recognised the disproportionate demands made by the Registered Homes Act 1984 on areas such as Kent where an unusually large number of private residential homes were encouraged by the abundance of dwellings suitable for conversion for this purpose. [4]

In practice, the likelihood of the emergence of an effective system of regulation for private and voluntary homes is difficult to determine. Indeed the present study gives rise to a number of important questions in this respect. The comparison of the Inner London Borough investigated here, and that of Kent, is useful for drawing attention to the problem of the variable impact of the Act. It seems important to determine the effect of the relationship between the number of homes involved in an authority's area, the level of payment for the registration service determined by DHSS, and the policy adopted towards residential care by the authority's social services department. Is it possible that in time, large demand for the service in an area such as Kent, will create a politically high profile for the service which will counteract any already established antipathy towards residential care at policy making and service delivery levels of the local authority? Will areas of heavy demand be able to take advantage of economies of scale to produce services of disproportionately high quality? In an area such as that with which the present study has been concerned, where there is a dearth of properties suitable for residential care accommodation, is it likely that low demand for the registration service will draw a weak response from policy makers which, together with no opportunities for economies of scale, will give rise to a low standard of service? Or will political hostility, particularly to the private market, in some areas such as these, ensure a vigilant response?

However, the present study demonstrates that the scale of demand and resources are not alone in determining standard of service. The demand on the registration services of the Borough were always relatively low, and it was precisely during the period of rapid increases in the level of funding for personal social services, particularly in cases where they were provided by inner city areas - 1971 to 1976 - that interest in the regulation of standards in the Home for the deaf evaporated.

In the absence of any real possibility that local authorities will be able to threaten de-registration and closure in the event of unsatisfactory standards in voluntary and private homes, they will have to fall back on persistent persuasion. At this point it is important to remember what is meant by satisfactory standards in this context: it is not the mere absence of physical or psychological abuse which is required, but a physical environment and a care regime which ensure for residents of private and voluntary homes fulfilment, dignity, autonomy, individuality, esteem, the satisfaction of emotional needs, and the normal range of choice and risk. And the code of practice associated with the Registered Homes Act details the means by which these objectives may be achieved. [5] That persistent persuasion may achieve much is evident from the history of the relationship between the Borough and the Home. Therefore, it is important to consider those features of that relationship before 1972, which seem to have been important as determinants of a policy of sustained intervention by the Borough in the affairs of the Charity.

It seems clear that a crucial role was played by the Registration Officer. Not only were her visits more frequent than the evidence suggests was generally the case, her reports were unusually thorough, detailed and lengthy, covering both the physical environment of the residents of the Home, as well as the care regime and its impact on residents. It is unclear from the evidence why this particular Registration Officer should have acted in such an atypical way. Perhaps the motivation was personal interest, perhaps an important factor was the interest of the Chief Welfare Officer. It is striking that the code of practice for registration authorities, while indicating that considerable qualities - personal, professional, and experiential - are required of those appointed as registration officers, nothing is said about their training. For example,

> Members of staff ... should be knowledgeable and skilled in communicating with proprietors from a wide range of backgrounds. They should have sufficient experience and status to receive the respect of colleagues and staff of homes alike. The demands made on officers engaged in this work are such that the registration officer should ensure that other, unrelated demands made on them are kept to a minimum. [6]

This suggests the necessity for the creation of a new specialism, a notion reinforced by the observation in the code that 'In at least one region of the county officers have set up an association which holds regular seminars and meetings. These are generally agreed to be beneficial. Other regions may well consider doing this.' [7]

In practice, field social workers appear to have some of the qualities required for the position - a knowledge of client groups likely to need residential care, and experience of dealing with a wide range of professionals from outside the field of the personal social services, such as those in health, education, and social security. However, a problem arises from the fact that field social workers tend not to have extensive experience of residential care: only a minority of residential workers have the CQSW. Typically, any experience of residential work tends to be short term and acquired before the CQSW is granted. Moreover, in terms of the professional social work hierarchy, promotion tends to be secured through the prestigious and politically sensitive area of child care. Thus, although the numbers of trained staff in residential settings, particularly those with the CSS are increasing, they do not yet represent a large pool from which future registration officers, already well regarded by colleagues, may be drawn. Furthermore, professional prestige tends to be associated, both for reasons of history (the failure of residential work to attract trained staff until recently), and skill (the range of diagnostic and treatment skills, particularly those based on methods derived from psychology and psychiatry) with work with children and families. Until the professional hierarchy is reversed, and the knowledge acquired through field social work is seen as an essential preparation for work in residential care, a setting in which people are at their most vulnerable, field social workers with post experience training involving both the practice and policy elements of residential care, which would include the financial management of homes would seem to be the most appropriate personnel from whom to make appointments to the post of registration officer. It seems reasonable, in the context of current circumstances, that such post experience training courses should be paid for out of the registration and inspection fees levied on voluntary and private homes. Ultimately, such courses could become the basis for the professionalisation of residential care work and the enhancement of its prestige. It seems likely that only such a development could ensure that statutory provision of residential care reaches the standards required of the voluntary and private sectors as set out in the code of practice.

A further problem associated with the reliance on field social work to supply personnel for the registration service is the growing, and in many ways de facto specialisation among trained social work staff. Although it is true that much specialisation, such as the concentration of trained field work staff in child care, and the reliance on occupational therapists to spearhead the development of services for the physically handicapped has resulted from an ad hoc response to general political pressures, in other cases it has emerged as a planned outcome of policy, as in the case of the increasing recruitment by local authorities of specialist workers for deaf and mentally handicapped people, as well as the mentally ill. In view of the fact that few social workers can be expected to understand the special requirements of all groups, a good registration service would require the registration officer's visits to be supplemented by those of the relevant specialist worker. Assessments of homes for registration purposes, and the monitoring of such homes, should be based on reports by both types of worker cooperating closely in the registration process. In the case of the Borough and the Home, the process by which improvements at the Home were secured before 1972 drew much of its strength from the involvement of the Deaf Specialist worker who operated in conjunction with the Registration Officer: because of the language barrier, only the Deaf Specialist was in a position to understand the nature of the relationship between the residents and the staff of the Home.

Even so, the effective regulation of private and voluntary homes will not be secured without clearly defined policies regarding the local authority's attitude to and use of such establishments, and the active involvement of the social services directorate in the assessment and monitoring process. A crucial element in the success of the Borough's role in encouraging improvements in the Home before 1972 was the fact that the Chief Welfare Officer was involved first, by receiving the reports of the Registration Officer and the Deaf Specialist; second, by helping to formulate policies regarding the Home; third, by checking that such policies were carried out; fourth, by intervening on behalf of his staff when they found his support necessary; and finally, by providing the point at which the buck stopped. It seems essential that it should be clear to everyone concerned that the principle that ultimate responsibility for the regulation of private and voluntary homes rests with the social services directorate, not the registration officer, is a reality.

Nevertheless, it must be admitted that in the case of the Home and the Borough, such factors produced a measure of success only because the Borough was able to persuade the Home's management committee of its point of view. The outcome would have been even more uncertain if a less compliant management committee had been involved. Certainly, the Borough's system of surveillance and persuasion would have been less effective in the event of a determinedly unscrupulous proprietor. In such circumstances, it may well be that interested pressure groups in the locality could provide a focus for community pressure, as happened in the case of the Home during the period from 1984. However, active pressure groups prepared to be assertive and politically adept at generating and publicising local concern are more numerous in inner city areas, where the opportunities for purchasing suitable properties for conversion to residential homes are most restricted. And, as we have seen from the history of the Borough and the Home, even a voluntary body, which, because of its charitable objectives, might be thought to be more likely than a commercial venture to succumb to popular pressure, may ignore hostile local reactions with impunity. For, while commercial ventures might not relish bad publicity, they would be able to ignore it for so long as the shortage of places in residential care continued.

In the short term, considerable hope must reside in the capacity of local authorities at least to check on proprietors of new homes to ensure that those previously guilty of running homes below registerable standard are not allowed to re-register or expand their provision of residential accommodation. In the long-term, however, one of the most effective ways of ensuring appropriate care practices would be to require those working in residential establishments, other than domestic staff, to have both a basic social work qualification and a post-experience training on a validated and designated course in residential care.

Thus from the point of view of local authorities, considerable difficulties attach to the task of ensuring that the registration of private and voluntary homes under the provisions of the Registered Homes Act 1984 is effective. However, equally considerable imponderables emerge from any consideration of the likely effect of the successful implementation of the Act on the supply of residential care. There is no question but that the standards operating in residential homes should be high to protect those who are dependent on others for shelter. Yet the costs of supplying those standards, in terms of buildings, facilities and staff, as well as of a regulation system, are bound to be considerable for the providers of residential care, and those costs will largely determine the price of the service. As we have seen, the dramatic upswing in the provision of residential care places outside the local authority sector arose from a deliberate attempt to encourage, and reinforce the existence of the mixed economy of welfare. The consequence was an immediate and unrestricted rise in the price of accommodation. The government panicked as the consequences for public expenditure levels threatened its economic strategy, and pegged the level at which it was prepared to subsidise places in accordance with that strategy. Neither of these actions, which had massive implications for the lives of thousands of vulnerable people, were determined by any reference to policy regarding the role of residential care in our society. Indeed, in so far as such a policy could be said to exist, the encouragement of residential care must be seen to be in clear contradiction to it: government social policy statements have emphasised the desirability of care in private households to depress the costs of care and to oblige families and neighbourhoods to stand on their own feet by responding to the needs of their members with as little recourse to dependency on the public purse as possible.

The dangers in human terms of acting according to broad ideological principles without reference to a policy on residential care became obvious when the decision to peg the levels of DHSS subsidy jeopardised the security of many residents in private and voluntary homes. If government is serious about the necessity for residential care and the necessity of securing good standards in private and voluntary homes, the level of subsidy must reflect the cost of those standards. If the economic consequences are unpalatable, then it seems likely that in the future good residential care will be available to those who can pay, while those who cannot will depend on ever-thinly spread 'community care'.

Appendix

The purpose of the table of events which follows is not to give details of the contents of the records for the period 1969 to 1983, but to provide a visual impression of the changing relationship between the Borough and the Home during those years as illustrated by the distribution over time of letters, memoranda, and so on, in the possession of the Borough, concerning the Home. The Table demonstrates the frequent interaction between Borough and Home during the period when promotional welfare was pursued by the Welfare Department's Chief Officer, through his Registration Officer for the Home, and his specialist Welfare Officer for the deaf, between 1969 and 1971.

With the demise of the Welfare Department, and the reorganisation of local authority personal social services into a single social services department, the interaction between Borough and Home declines, especially when responsibility for the Home is devolved to an Area Office. The change in the relationship, which is apparent in 1973, becomes marked in 1974, and interaction between the Home and the Borough dwindles dramatically until June 1978, when the Home's financial predicament prompts the Management Committee to seek the help of the Social Services Directorate by engaging in a discussion about the future role of the Home.

However, the flurry of interest in the Home is short-lived. Between June and October 1978, correspondence concerning the Home is striking in its quantity compared with the previous four years. But thereafter, despite being fully informed about the Home's financial situation, and the anxieties of the Management Committee about its future, no initiative regarding the Home is taken by the Borough's Social Services Directorate. Indeed, during the years 1979, 1981, 1982 and 1983, the dearth of correspondence in the records is eloquent testimony to the Borough's lack of interest in the Home. It is not until the Autumn of 1984, when the Home's very existence is in question, that the Directorate is forced to pay attention to the Home once more.

TABLE OF EVENTS

The Borough and Home 1969 to 1983

1969

January.

1. 9 January - Visit by Registration Officer and specialist Welfare Officer recorded by specialist Welfare Officer.
2. Registration schedule completed by Registration Officer.

February.

1. 3 February - Chief Welfare Officer of an Outer London Borough thanks the Borough for the report on one of the residents it sponsors at the Home.
2. 10 February - Chief Welfare Officer of Borough sends report to his counterpart in a West Country County on one of the residents sponsored by that County at the Home.
3. Chief Welfare Officer tells Matron that fundraising walkers are to visit the Home.

March.

1. 3 March - Chairman of Management Committee to Chief Welfare Officer concerning arrangements at new Day Centre.
2. 19 March - Chief Welfare Officer to Matron clarifying arrangements at the Day Centre.
3. 19 March - Chief Welfare Officer to Chairman of Management Committee clarifying arrangements at the Day Centre.

April.

1. 21 April - Chief Welfare Officer of an outer London borough asks the Borough to check up on and report on two of the Home's residents whom it sponsors.
2. 30 April - Management Committee telephones asking for advice about the kind of person to be appointed assistant matron.
3. Copy of proposed advert for assistant matron.

May.

June.

1. 11 June - Chief Welfare Officer to Chairman of Management Committee with suggested advert for assistant Matron.

July.

1. 15 July - Registration reinspection report.
2. Charity's Annual Report and Accounts.
3. Note by Registration Officer about what needs to be done to improve Home.
4. 28 July - letter from Chief Welfare Officer to Management Committee concerning required improvements.
5. 31 July - Chief Welfare Officer to counterpart in a County reporting on sponsored resident's social activities.
6. 31 July - Chairman of Management Committee to Chief Welfare Officer concerning new Matron.

August.

1. 6 August - Chief Welfare Officer to Management Committee - new Matron, therefore there must be new registration.
2. 8 August - Open Day at the Home attended by the Mayor of the Borough.
3. 14 August - County Chief Welfare Officer thanks Borough for information on residents.

September.

1. 4 September - Chairman of Management Committee to Chief Welfare Officer concerning registration and new Matron.

October.

1. 21 October - Chief Welfare Officer to Matron concerning

Day Centre arrangements.

2. 31 October - Chief Welfare Officer to Matron concerning Christmas shopping expedition.

November.

December.

1. 9 December - New registration schedule completed by Registration Officer.
2. 9 December - Report on his visit by the specialist Welfare Officer.

1970

January.

February.

1. 5 February - note - new Matron having difficulty sorting out the accounts.
2. Query from the Chief Welfare Officer regarding residents' financial contributions.

March.

April.

May.

1. 5 May - Chief Welfare Officer to Matron - new registration required.

June.

July.

August.

1. 25 August - Registration Officer completes new registration schedule.

September.

October.

November.

1. 9 November - Chief Welfare Officer to Matron regarding Christmas shopping expedition.
2. 11 November - Matron sends thanks and tells of new assistant.
3. 19 November - Chief Welfare Officer to Matron requesting names for shopping expedition.

December.

1971

January.

February.

1. 17 February - Matron to specialist Welfare Officer asking

for help in finding suitable alternative holiday accommodation.

2. Chief Welfare Officer offers Matron the use of the Borough's holiday hotel.

March.

1. 11 March - Matron thanks Chief Welfare Officer and reports on plans for redecoration.
2. 24 March - Chief Welfare Officer to his counterparts who sponsored residents at the Home about the costs of the holiday.
3. 26 March - Chief Welfare Officer about works to be done at the Home.
4. 31 March - GLC Architects Dept to Chief Welfare Officer about fire precautions at the Home.
5. During March letters from other Welfare Departments regarding the costs of residents' holidays.

April.

1. 26 April - Matron to Chief Welfare Officer to report that all but one of the works had been carried out, and the remainder would be done during the holiday.
2. Chief Welfare Officer to Matron to say that all other Departments had agreed to pay for the holidays.

May.

June.

1. 7 June - Report by Registration Officer on reinspection visit.
2. Matron thanks Chief Welfare Officer for holiday.
3. 13 June - Matron confers with Chief Welfare Officer about residents and clubs etc.
4. 30 June - Chief Welfare Officer clarifies situation with Matron regarding the clubs.

July.

August.

September.

1. 28 September - Enquiry from a County to discover whether Home suitable for 21 years old woman.
2. 30 September - reply about the nature of the Home.
3. Receipt of letters from Departments outside Borough asking for reports on the residents whom they were sponsoring.

October.

November.

December.

1972

January.

1. 20 January - Completion of reinspection schedule by Registration Officer.

February.

March.

April.

May.

1. Letters to other Welfare Departments regarding holidays for residents.
2. All Welfare Departments give permission.
3. 9 May - Chairman of Management Committee seeks help from Director of Social Services for help with payment for adaptations.

June.

1. Senior Social Worker signs letters regarding holidays.
2. 27 June - Chairman of Management Committee to Director concerning finance.

July.

1. 4 July - Auditor declares Home's finance arrangements acceptable.

August.

September.

October.

November.

December.

1973

January.

February.

1. 15 February - Matron to Associate Director thanking him for arranging art classes.
2. 20 February - Visit to Home by Voluntary Homes Inspector - report.

March.

April.

May.

1. 14 May - short report from Home's Inspector to outer London borough on their residents in the Home.
2. 22 May - a county reports that it will not pay automatically for its residents' holidays.

June.

July.

1. 13 July - Management Committee asks to raise the maintenance fee to help pay for the adaptations needed.
2. Rise agreed.

August.

September.

October.

November.

December.

1974

January.

February.

March.

1. 12 March - letter regarding the maintenance of one resident.

April.

May.

June.

1. 12 June - Hand-written note for report to outer London borough regarding the Home and one of the residents sponsored by the borough.

July.

August.

September.

October.

November.

December.

1975

January.

February.

March.

April.

May.

June.

July.

August.

September.

1. 19 September - Chairman of the Management Committee to the Director of Social Services suggesting maintenance fees be raised to pay for adaptations.

October.

1. 20 October - Director of Social Services agrees to the fees being raised.

November.

December.

1976

January.

February.

March.

April.

May.

June.

1. 1 June - Borough Accountant agrees to loan to Charity and the raising of the maintenance fee.
2. 10 June - Letter to Chairman of the Management Committee confirming the loan of £12,500.

July.

August.

September.

October.

November.

December.

1977

January.

February.

March.

April.

May.

June.

July.

1. 27 July - Report of GLC Architects Department on the home.

August.

September.

October.

1. 29 October - Invitation to Director of Social Services to attend the Charity's Annual General Meeting, which is declined.

November.

December.

1978

January.

February.

March.

April.

May.

June.

1. 1 June - Invitation to Director to lunch with the Chairman of the Management Committee to discuss the future of the Home.
2. 6 June - note from Director to suggest a meeting after lunch.
3. 7 June - Director makes firm appointment to see Chairman of Management Committee.
4. 28 June - New registration - registration report schedule completed by Registration Officer.

July.

1. 4 July - Director writes to London Directors asking about the possible uses to which the Home might be put.
2. Chairman of the Management Committee to Director reporting on the cost of upgrading the fire arrangements to satisfy the GLC and asking for a loan of £10,000.
3. 27 July - reply from an outer London borough concerning the Director's request for information on the future use of the Home.

August.

1. 8 August - Reply from London Borough on future of the Home.
2. 15 August - Reply from London Borough unable to respond about future of the Home because they have no deaf specialist worker on staff.
3. 17 August - Reply from inner London borough on future of the Home.
4. 29 August - Reply from outer London borough on future of the Home.

September.

1. 1 September - Reply from London Borough on future of the Home.
2. 4 September - Reply from outer London Borough on future of the Home.
3. Reply from outer London borough on future of Home.

October.

1. 6 October - Reply from Director to inner London borough concerning future of Home.
2. 6 October - Director sends Chairman of the Management Committee an analysis of the replies from the London boroughs on the future of the Home.

November.

December.

1979

January.

February.

March.

April.

May.

June.

1. 11 June - Letter from Matron because she is worried about the number of cancellations of visits to the Day Centre in the last six weeks.
2. 18 June - Reply to Matron informing her that the problem is one of transport.
3. 28 June - Day Care to Matron to report the acquisition of two additional vehicles.

July.

August.

September.

October.

November.

December.

1980

January.

February.

March.

April.

May.

June.

July.

August.

September.

October.

November.

December.

1981

January.

February.

March.

April.

May.

June.

July.

August.

September.

October.

November.

December.

1982

January.

February.

March.

1. 12 March - Letter regarding the cost of holidays.

April.

May.

June.

July.

August.

September.

October.

November.

December.

1983

January.

February.

March.

April.

May.

June.

July.

August.

September.

October.

November.

December.

Bibliography

Abel, R.A.D., An Investigation into some Aspects of Visual Handicap, Statistical and Research Report, Series no. 14, HMSO, London, 1976.

Abel, R.A.D., 'The identification and registration of the blind, 1834-1968', unpublished PhD thesis, London School of Economics and Political Science, University of London, 1987.

Abel-Smith, B. and Titmuss, R.M., The Cost of the National Health Service in England and Wales, Cambridge University Press, Cambridge, 1956.

Abel-Smith, B., Value for Money in Health Services, Heinemann, London, 1977.

Abrams, P., 'Realities of neighbourhood care', Policy and Politics, vol. 12, no. 4, 1984.

Advisory Council for Hearing Impaired People, Report of a Sub-Committee appointed to consider the Role of Social Services in the Care of the Deaf of all Ages, DHSS, London, June 1977.

Bacon, R., and Eltis, W., Britain's Economic Problems: Too Few

Producers, Macmillan, London, 1976.

Barton, R., Institutional Neurosis, John Wright, 1959.

Bayley, M., Mental Handicap and Community Care, Routledge and Kegan Paul, London, 1973.

Becker, G., Growing Old in Silence, University of California Press, 1980.

Booth, T., Home Truths - Old People's Homes and the Outcome of Care, Gower, Aldershot, 1985.

Bowlby, J., Maternal Care and Mental Health, World Health Organisation, Geneva, 1952.

Brown, M., 'The development of local authority welfare services 1948 to 1965 under Part Three of the National Assistance Act 1948', unpublished PhD thesis, Manchester, 1972.

Bulmer, M., Neighbours: the Work of Philip Abrams, Cambridge University Press, 1986.

Bulmer, M., The Social Basis of Community Care, Allen and Unwin, 1987.

Bunting, C., Public Attitudes to Deafness, OPCS, HMSO, London, 1981.

Camden, London Borough of, 'Independent review of residential care for the elderly within the London Borough of Camden', unpublished report, 1987.

Centre for Policy on Aging, Home Life: a code of practice for residential care, London, 1984.

Clough, R., Beyond Barclay: the future of residential care, Social Care Association, 1981.

Community Care, 21 January 1988, pp. 1 and 5.

Conrad, R., The Deaf School Child, Harper and Row, London, 1979.

Consultative Group on the Law and the Rights of Vulnerable Elderly People, The Law and Vulnerable Elderly People, Age Concern, 1986.

Cooper, J., The Creation of the British Personal Social

Services 1962 - 74, Heinemann, London, 1983.

DHSS, Priorities in Health and Personal Social Services in England, HMSO, London, 1976.

DHSS, Forward Planning for Local Authority Social Services, Circular LASSL, (77) 13, 1977.

Deuchar, M., 'Diglossia in British Sign Language', PhD Dissertation, Stanford University, 1978.

Donnison, D., Jay, P., and Stewart, M., The Ingleby Report: Three Critical Essays, Fabian Research Series 231, London, 1962.

Duckworth, D., The Classification and Measurement of Disablement, DHSS, Research Report No. 10, HMSO, London, 1983.

Glennerster, H., 'The wilting flowers of community care', Community Care, September 12, 1985.

Goffman, E., Assylums: essays on the social situations of mental patients and other inmates, Anchor Books, New York 196

Goldberg, E.M. and Hatch S. (eds), A New Look at the Personal Social Services, Discussion Paper No. 4, PSI, London, 1981.

Gough, I., The Political Economy of the Welfare State, Macmillan, London, 1979.

Hall, P., Reforming the Welfare: the politics of change in the personal social services, Heinemann, London, 1976.

Hatch, S., Outside the State, Croom Helm, London, 1980.

Home Office, The Child, the Family, and the Young Offender, Cmnd. 2742, HMSO, London, 1965.

Home Office, Children in Trouble, Cmnd. 3601, HMSO, London, 1968.

Jones, D., and Mayo, M., Community Work One, Routledge and Kegan Paul, London, 1974.

Jones, D., and Mayo, M., Community Work Two, Routledge and Kegan Paul, London, 1975.

Kramer, J., and Piachaud, D., 'The micro-economics of old

people's homes', British Journal of Social Work, 12, 1982, pp. 171-187.

Keeble, U., Aids and Adaptations, Occasional Papers on Social Administration, no. 62, Bedford Square Press, London, 1979.

Kin, R., Raynes M., and Tizard, J., Patterns of Residential Care, Routledge and Kegan Paul, London, 1971.

Marshall, T.H., Social Policy in the Twentieth Century, Hutchinson, London, 1975.

Ministry of Health, A Hospital Plan for England and Wales, Cmnd. 1604, HMSO, London, 1962.

Health and Welfare: the development of community care, Cmnd. 1973, HMSO, London, 1963.

National Institute for Social Work, Residential Care: a positive choice, HMSO, London, 1988.

Owens, P., Community and Severe Physical Disability, Occasional Papers on Social Administration, no. 82, Bedford Square Press, London, 1987.

Reddin, M., Universality and Selectivity: strategies in social policy, National Economic and Social Council (Eire) Report no. 36, Dublin, 1977.

Reddin, M., 'Occupation Welfare and Social Division' in Jones, C., and Stevenson, J. (eds), Yearbook of Social Policy in Britain, 1980-81, Routledge and Kegan Paul, London, 1982.

Regulations under Registered Homes Act 1984, Statutory Instrument no. 1345, 1984.

Report of the Royal Commission on the Law Relating to Mental Illness and Mental Deficiency, HMSO, Cmnd. 169, London, 1957.

Report of the Committee on Children and Young Persons, Cmnd. 1191, HMSO, London, 1960.

Report of the Committee of Inquiry into Allegations of Ill-treatment of Patients and other Irregularities at the Ely Hospital, Cardiff, National Health Service, Cmnd. 3975, HMSO, London, 1969.

Report of the Committee on Local Authority and Allied Personal Social Services, Cmnd. 3703, HMSO, London, 1969.

Robb, R., Sans Everything: a case to answer, Nelson, London, 1967.

Rodgers, B. and Dixon, J., A Portrait of Social Work, Oxford University Press, 1960.

Roof, M., A Hundred Years of Family Welfare, Michael Joseph, London, 1972.

Rosser, C., and Harris, C., The Family and Social Change, Routledge and Kegan Paul, London, 1965.

Royal Commission on Local Government in Greater London, 1957-1960, Cmnd. 1164, HMSO, London, 1960.

Sainsbury, S., Registered as Disabled, Occasional Papers on Social Administration no. 35, Bell, London, 1970.

Sainsbury, S., Measuring Disability, Occasional Papers on Social Administration no. 54, 1973.

Sainsbury, S., Deaf Worlds, Hutchinson, London, 1986.

Social Policy Research, The Implementation of the Chronically Sick and Disabled Persons Act 1970, Social Policy Research Ltd.

Sorsby, A., The Incidence and Causes of Blindness in England and Wales, 1963-1968, DHSS, HMSO, London, 1972.

Stevenson, S., Specialisation and Social Service Teams, George Allen and Unwin, London, 1981.

The Registered Homes Act 1984: Guidance for Registration, London Boroughs Working Party, First Edition, Croydon, May 1985.

Titmuss, R.M., Income Distribution and Social Change, George Allen and Unwin, London, 1962.

Topliss, E., and Gould, B., A Charter for the Disabled, Basil Blackwell and Martin Robertson, London, 1981.

Townsend, P., The Family Life of Old People, Routledge and Kegan Paul, London, 1957.

Townsend, P., The Last Refuge, Routledge and Kegal Paul, London, 196

Townsend, P., 'Introduction' in Morris, P., Put Away, Routledge and Kegan Paul, London, 1969.

Webb, A., Day, L., and Weller, D., Voluntary Social Services Manpower Resources, Personal Social Services Council, 1976.

Wilmott, P., and Young, M., Family and Kinship in East London, Routledge and Kegan Paul, London, 1957.

Wilmott, P., and Young, M., Family and Class in a London Suburb, Routledge and Kegan Paul, London, 1960.

Wilmott, P., Social Networks, Informal Care and Public Policy, Research Report 655, PSI, London, 1986.

Wolfenden, J., The Future of Voluntary Organisations, Croom Helm, London, 1977.

Younghusband, E., Report of the Working Party on Social Workers in the Local Authority Health and Welfare Services, HMSO, London, 1959.